Artificial Intelligence in the Clinical Laboratory: Current Practice and Emerging Opportunities

Editor

JASON M. BARON

CLINICS IN LABORATORY MEDICINE

www.labmed.theclinics.com

Consulting Editor
MILENKO JOVAN TANASIJEVIC

March 2023 • Volume 43 • Number 1

ELSEVIER

1600 John F. Kennedy Boulevard • Suite 1800 • Philadelphia, Pennsylvania, 19103-2899

http://www.theclinics.com

CLINICS IN LABORATORY MEDICINE Volume 43, Number 1
March 2023 ISSN 0272-2712, ISBN-13: 978-0-323-93983-6

Editor: Taylor Hayes
Developmental Editor: Ann Gielou M. Posedio

Reprints. For copies of 100 or more, of articles in this publication, please contact the Commercial Reprints Department, Elsevier Inc., 360 Park Avenue South, New York, New York 10010-1710. Tel. 212-633-3874, Fax: 212-633-3820, E-mail: reprints@elsevier.com.

Clinics in Laboratory Medicine (ISSN 0272-2712) is published quarterly by Elsevier Inc., 360 Park Avenue South, New York, NY 10010-1710. Months of issue are March, June, September, and December. Business and Editorial offices: 1600 John F. Kennedy Blvd., Suite 1800, Philadelphia, PA 19103-2899. Periodicals postage paid at New York, NY and additional mailing offices. Subscription prices are $291.00 per year (US individuals), $657.00 per year (US institutions), $100.00 per year (US students), $374.00 per year (Canadian individuals), $798.00 per year (Canadian institutions), $100.00 per year (Canadian students), $416.00 per year (international individuals), $798.00 per year (international institutions), $185.00 (international students). Foreign air speed delivery is included in all Clinics subscription prices. All prices are subject to change without notice. POSTMASTER: Send address changes to *Clinics in Laboratory Medicine*, Elsevier Health Sciences Division, Subscription Customer Service, 3251 Riverport Lane, Maryland Heights, MO 63043. **Customer Service: 1-800-654-2452 (US). From outside of the US and Canada, call 1-314-447-8871. Fax: 1-314-447-8029. E-mail: journalscustomerservice-usa@elsevier.com (for print support) or journalsonlinesupport-usa@elsevier.com (for online support).**

Clinics in Laboratory Medicine is covered in *EMBASE/Exerpta Medica, MEDLINE/PubMed (Index Medicus), Cinahl, Current Contents/Clinical Medicine, BIOSIS* and *ISI/BIOMED.*

Contributors

EDITOR-IN-CHIEF

MILENKO JOVAN TANASIJEVIC, MD, MBA
Vice Chair for Clinical Pathology and Quality, Department of Pathology, Director of Clinical Laboratories, Brigham and Women's Hospital, Dana-Farber Cancer Institute, Associate Professor of Pathology, Harvard Medical School, Boston, Massachusetts, USA

EDITOR

JASON M. BARON, MD
Assistant Professor, Part Time, Department of Pathology, Massachusetts General Hospital, Harvard Medical School, Boston, Massachusetts, USA

AUTHORS

JASON M. BARON, MD
Assistant Professor, Part Time, Department of Pathology, Massachusetts General Hospital, Harvard Medical School, Boston, Massachusetts, USA

DUSTIN R. BUNCH, PhD
Department of Pathology and Laboratory Medicine, Nationwide Children's Hospital, Department of Pathology, College of Medicine, The Ohio State University, Columbus, Ohio, USA

JOHN KIM CHOI, MD, PhD
Division of Laboratory Medicine, The University of Alabama at Birmingham, WP P230N, Birmingham, Alabama, USA

SHIMUL CHOWDHURY, PhD
Rady Children's Institute for Genomic Medicine, San Diego, California, USA

ANAND S. DIGHE, MD, PhD
Associate Professor, Department of Pathology, Massachusetts General Hospital, Harvard Medical School, Boston, Massachusetts, USA

THOMAS J.S. DURANT, MD
Department of Laboratory Medicine, Yale School of Medicine, New Haven, Connecticut, USA

ASHLEY EMMONS, MS
Roche Diagnostics, Indianapolis, Indiana, USA

DENISE L. HEANEY, PhD
Roche Diagnostics, Indianapolis, Indiana, USA

ALISON HELLMANN, BS
Roche Diagnostics, Indianapolis, IN, USA

KIELY N. JAMES, PhD
Genomics, Rady Children's Institute for Genomic Medicine, San Diego, California, USA

JAMES L. JANUZZI JR, MD
Department of Medicine, Division of Cardiology, Massachusetts General Hospital, Department of Medicine, Division of Cardiology, Harvard Medical School, Baim Institute for Clinical Research, Boston, Massachusetts, USA

DANIELLE E. KURANT, MD
Research Fellow, Medical Oncology, Dana-Farber Cancer Institute, Harvard Medical School, Boston, Massachusetts, USA

MATTHEW B.A. MCDERMOTT, PhD
Postdoctoral Researcher, CSAIL, MIT, Cambridge, Massachusetts, USA

PAUL E. MEAD, PhD, SCYM(ASCP)
Department of Pathology, St. Jude Children's Research Hospital, Memphis, Tennessee, USA

SAM A. MICHELHAUGH, BA
Georgetown University School of Medicine, Washington, DC, USA

BRET NESTOR, MS
PhD Student, Department of Computer Science, University of Toronto, Toronto, Canada

KETAN PARANJAPE, PhD, MBA
Roche Diagnostics, Indianapolis, Indiana, USA

SUJAL PHADKE, PhD
Genomics, Rady Children's Institute for Genomic Medicine, San Diego, California, USA

JOSEPH W. RUDOLF, MD
Department of Pathology, University of Utah School of Medicine, ARUP Laboratories, Salt Lake City, Utah, USA

MATTHEW STEWART PRIME, BSC, MBBS, PhD, MRCS(ENG)
Roche Information Solutions, Riehen, Basel Stadt, Switzerland

PETER SZOLOVITS, PhD
Professor of Computer Science and Engineering, CSAIL, MIT, Cambridge, Massachusetts, USA

TERENCE C. WONG, PhD
Genomics, Rady Children's Institute for Genomic Medicine, San Diego, California, USA

Contents

> This article provides an overview of machine learning fundamentals and some applications of machine learning to clinical laboratory diagnostics and patient management. A key goal of this article is to provide a basic foundation in clinical machine learning for readers with clinical laboratory experience that will set them up for more in-depth study of the topic and/or to become a better collaborator with computational colleagues in the development and deployment of machine learning–based solutions.

> Laboratory clinical decision support (CDS) typically relies on data from the electronic health record (EHR). The implementation of a sustainable, effective laboratory CDS program requires a commitment to standardization and harmonization of key EHR data elements that are the foundation of laboratory CDS. The direct use of artificial intelligence algorithms in CDS programs will be limited unless key elements of the EHR are structured. The identification, curation, maintenance, and preprocessing steps necessary to implement robust laboratory-based algorithms must account for the heterogeneity of data present in a typical EHR.

> Clinical artificial intelligence (AI)/machine learning (ML) is anticipated to offer new abilities in clinical decision support, diagnostic reasoning, precision medicine, clinical operational support, and clinical research, but careful concern is needed to ensure these technologies work effectively in the clinic. Here, we detail the clinical ML/AI design process, identifying several key questions and detailing several common forms of issues that arise with ML tools, as motivated by real-world examples, such that clinicians and researchers can better anticipate and correct for such issues in their own use of ML/AI techniques

> Artificial intelligence (AI) applications are an area of active investigation in clinical chemistry. Numerous publications have demonstrated the promise of AI across all phases of testing including preanalytic, analytic, and

postanalytic phases; this includes novel methods for detecting common specimen collection errors, predicting laboratory results and diagnoses, and enhancing autoverification workflows. Although AI applications pose several ethical and operational challenges, these technologies are expected to transform the practice of the clinical chemistry laboratory in the near future.

Artificial intelligence (AI) is becoming an indispensable tool to augment decision making in different health care settings and by various members of the patient pathway, including the patient. AI provides the ability to optimize data to bring clinical decision support for clinicians and laboratorians and/or empower patients to actively participate in their own health care. Though there are many examples of AI in health care, the exact role of AI and digital health solutions is still taking shape. Although AI will not replace the clinician, those who do not adopt AI may in time, be left behind.

The development of artificial intelligence and machine learning algorithms may allow for advances in patient care. There are existing and potential applications in cancer diagnosis and monitoring, identification of at-risk groups of individuals, classification of genetic variants, and even prediction of patient ancestry. This article provides an overview of some current and future applications of artificial intelligence in genomic medicine, in addition to discussing challenges and considerations when bringing these tools into clinical practice.

Advancements in technology have improved biomarker discovery in the field of heart failure (HF). What was once a slow and laborious process has gained efficiency through use of high-throughput omics platforms to phenotype HF at the level of genes, transcripts, proteins, and metabolites. Furthermore, improvements in artificial intelligence (AI) have made the interpretation of large omics data sets easier and improved analysis. Use of omics and AI in biomarker discovery can aid clinicians by identifying markers of risk for developing HF, monitoring care, determining prognosis, and developing druggable targets. Combined, AI has the power to improve HF patient care.

Minimal residual disease detection provides critical prognostic predictor of treatment outcome and is the standard of care for B lymphoblastic leukemia. Flow cytometry–based minimal residual disease detection is the most common test modality and has high sensitivity (0.01%) and a rapid turnaround time (24 hours). This article details the leukemia associated immunophenotype analysis approach for flow cytometry–based minimal residual disease detection used at St. Jude Children's Research Hospital and importance of using guide gates and back-gating.

Kiely N. James, Sujal Phadke, Terence C. Wong and Shimul Chowdhury

The use of Natural Language Processing (NLP) and Artificial Intelligence (AI) have been introduced into various areas of medicine with the hopes of eliminating human bias, increasing accuracy, and efficiently deploying the medical workforce. With the incorporation of whole exome sequencing (WES) and whole genome sequencing (WGS) into the clinical setting in recent years, NLP and AI tools have been developed to help support the extensive manual effort required to analyze large amounts of genomic data. This chapter will summarize current tools and approaches of NLP and AI, and provide examples of how these tools can aid in the scalability and application of genomic medicine into clinical practice.

CLINICS IN LABORATORY MEDICINE

SERIES OF RELATED INTEREST

Advances in Molecular Pathology
Available at: https://www.journals.elsevier.com/advances-in-molecular-pathology

---

THE CLINICS ARE NOW AVAILABLE ONLINE!
Access your subscription at:
www.theclinics.com

Preface

Artificial Intelligence in the Clinical Laboratory

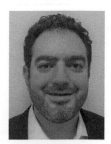

Jason M. Baron, MD
Editor

Artificial intelligence (AI) has become ubiquitous in many areas outside of health care with application so wide-ranging to include agricultural decision making, smartphone navigation, e-mail spam detection, predictive text, targeted marketing, environmental protection, criminal sentencing, employee hiring, and robotics among thousands of others. Clinical practice lags behind many other areas in terms of AI adoption, still relying primarily on manual human decision making. Nonetheless, clinical AI development and adoption are progressing and are poised to play a central role in many aspects of clinical practice in future decades, if not sooner. Indeed, AI is already integral to mission critical processes in some clinical laboratories. Thus, it is essential that pathologists, laboratorians, and others in health care gain at least a basic understanding of AI.

For example, clinical laboratory directors must make decisions about which tests to include on their laboratory's send-out test menus; in recent times, this responsibility has grown to include decisions about multianalyte assays with algorithmic analyses (MAAAs). MAAAs are often based on machine-learning algorithms, a subset of AI. Likewise, anatomic pathologists may be called upon to evaluate whether new digital histopathology image analysis systems and accompanying AI-based algorithms are well-suited to use in their clinical practices. While effectively evaluating these technologies may not require a detailed understanding of the machine learning algorithms underlying the MAAA or the image analysis system, having at least a basic understanding of machine learning and particularly well-known pitfalls may be vital. Moreover, pathologists and laboratorians can serve as invaluable collaborators and domain experts in developing and implementing new AI-based technologies; having at least a basic understanding of AI and the process of algorithm development will enable them to collaborate much more effectively.

Clin Lab Med 43 (2023) ix–x
https://doi.org/10.1016/j.cll.2022.09.001
0272-2712/23/© 2022 Published by Elsevier Inc.
labmed.theclinics.com

A key goal of this issue is to provide pathologists, laboratorians, and others within health care with a background in AI to enable them to (i) strategically evaluate and adopt new technologies; (ii) effectively collaborate in algorithm development initiatives; and (iii) have a strong foundation for more in-depth study of the topic. While this issue alone will not maximally achieve all these objectives, I hope that it will offer a very useful starting point.

Jason M. Baron, MD
Department of Pathology
Massachusetts General Hospital
Harvard Medical School
55 Fruit Street
Boston, MA 02114-2696, USA

E-mail address:
jmbaron@partners.org

Artificial Intelligence in the Clinical Laboratory

An Overview with Frequently Asked Questions

Jason M. Baron, MD

KEYWORDS

- Machine learning • Artificial intelligence • Clinical decision support
- Multianalyte assay with algorithmic analysis • Predictive model • Clinical laboratory

KEY POINTS

- Machine learning and artificial intelligence, commonplace in many areas outside of health care, offer tremendous potential to transform many aspects of laboratory diagnosis.
- Understanding fundamentals of machine learning will enable pathologists and other laboratorians to better evaluate tests and technologies for use in their laboratory and to better collaborate on projects involving predictive algorithm development, validation, and implementation.
- Machine learning projects often involves steps including (1) problem conception and development; (2) data extraction, cleaning, and assembly; (3) model training and model validation; and (4) model implementation.
- Clinical implementation of machine learning models requires addressing technical, administrative, evidentiary, and educational challenges.

INTRODUCTION

Laboratory medicine has traditionally relied mostly on manual clinician decision-making to select which laboratory tests to order and to apply laboratory test results to patient diagnosis and management.[1,2] However, modern machine learning approaches that are commonplace in many industries besides health care are poised to augment—and to some extent have already augmented—human decision-making in this realm with multiple benefits both to patients and clinicians.[2–6] Although this Clinics in Laboratory Medicine issue as a whole reviews a variety of laboratory artificial intelligence (AI) applications, strategies, and considerations in depth, this particular article is meant to provide a general foundation. This article, written mostly in question-and-answer format, looks at fundamentals of machine learning and

Department of Pathology, Massachusetts General Hospital, Harvard Medical School, 55 Fruit Street, Boston, MA 02114-2696, USA
E-mail address: jmbaron@partners.org

Clin Lab Med 43 (2023) 1–16
https://doi.org/10.1016/j.cll.2022.09.002
0272-2712/23/© 2023 Elsevier Inc. All rights reserved.

applications to medicine and provides a practical overview of the process of developing a clinical prediction model.

What is Artificial Intelligence and How Does This Differ from Machine Learning?

AI has varying definitions. Under the broadest definition virtually any software application that automates human tasks, supports human decision-making, or uses logic to mimic any aspect of human intelligence would be considered AI. Machine learning, discussed in much greater detail throughout this article, includes a class of algorithms that use "training" data to "learn" how to perform a task. Although machine learning is technically a subclass of AI, in common parlance, and as used throughout the remainder of this article, AI and machine learning are used interchangeably. For example, most currently deployed clinical decision support uses rule-based logic to advise or alert clinicians; this might be considered AI under a broad definition. However, in practice, this article and most informaticians would only consider clinical decision support to be "artificially intelligent" if based on machine learning.

What is Supervised Machine Learning and How Does It Differ from Unsupervised?

Machine learning can be divided into supervised, unsupervised, semisupervised, and reinforcement learning. Many clinical and research machine learning tasks use supervised machine learning. The goal of supervised machine learning is to predict the value of a target (dependent) variable from a set of predictors (also known as features). For example, suppose we want to predict whether a patient has sepsis based on patient vital signs and laboratory test results. We could use supervised machine learning; in this case, the target would be whether the patient has sepsis and the predictors would be the vital signs and test results.

The key defining attribute of supervised, as opposed to unsupervised, machine learning is that supervised machine learning starts with a set of *labeled* training data; that is, the training data contains ground truth values for the target variable in each case. Using the sepsis example, the labels would denote whether each patient in the training data set has sepsis. Once trained, a supervised machine learning model can predict the target variable for new cases where the value of the target variable is unknown. For example, the hypothetical sepsis model might be applied to a new patient, arriving at the emergency department with unknown sepsis status; in this case, the model would use the patient's test results and vital signs to predict whether the patient in fact has sepsis.

Unsupervised machine learning seeks to find patterns within data but does not require ground truth labels; similarly unsupervised machine learning does not directly predict a specific fundamental attribute within the data. Unsupervised machine learning is often used alone or in combination with supervised machine learning, particularly when identification of ground truth labels is difficult or costly. (Often curating ground truth labels can be among the most challenging aspects of a project; this article subsequently discusses strategies for ground truth curation). Unsupervised models typically take the form of clustering or dimensionality reduction. For example, we might use unsupervised machine learning to cluster patients by patterns of laboratory test results. Semisupervised machine learning uses primarily unlabeled but limited amounts of labeled data; generally, semisupervised learning would be useful in projects that require a supervised machine learning–like task (predict a target variable), but where labeled training data are limited and unlabeled training data are plentiful. Suppose, for example, a manual chart review was required for ground truth label curation in a given project. In this case, the research team might have access to considerably more patient data than they would have the resources to label and thus the project might lend itself well to semisupervised learning. Reinforcement learning is a third type of machine learning. Reinforcement learning has been used for tasks such as mastery of games (eg, the computer learns how to play chess by playing against itself millions or billions of times) and in robotics.

What is Classification and How Does It Differ from Regression?

Supervised machine learning is often applied to regression and classification tasks. Classification involves predicting a binary or categorical outcome. The previously mentioned hypothetical sepsis prediction model might be framed as binary classification with 2 outcomes: sepsis or no sepsis. Likewise, a classification model could predict multiple categories, for example, a model designed to take an image of a white blood cell and determine the cell type (lymphocyte, neutrophil, eosinophil, and so forth)

Although the final output of a classification model may be transformed to a single binary or categorical result (eg, cell is a neutrophil or patient has sepsis), most models generate probabilities of each class (eg, 87% chance the patient has sepsis). These probabilities can then be compared with a threshold to arrive at the ultimate classification. For example, we might trigger an alert if the sepsis model predicts the probability of sepsis greater than 25% threshold. By varying the threshold probabilities, model developers can tradeoff sensitivity versus specificity. For example, classifying patients as having sepsis if the predicted probability is greater than 25% would produce a more sensitive but less specific model than using a cutoff of 50%.

In contrast to classification, regression models predict numeric or ordinal outcomes. For example, a regression model might predict a patient's high-density lipoprotein cholesterol level (numerical result) or tumor grade (ordinal result).

What are Some Common Applications of Laboratory Artificial Intelligence?

In a general sense, laboratory AI can

1. Automate tasks that people would otherwise have to do but would rather not and
2. Perform tasks that would be impossible for people to do unaided.

An example of task automation is automated pathology image analysis. For example, some laboratories use machine learning–based image analysis to assist in "manual" white blood cell differentials.[7] Here, the main value of the AI is to reduce manual labor, thereby improving efficiency and freeing people for other less easily automated tasks. In contrast, other AI applications do not seek to replicate human tasks but rather perform tasks that would be impossible for people, for example, identifying complex genotype-phenotype relationships or predicting individualized patient survival.[8]

In developing algorithms designed to automate tasks previously performed by people, human annotation is often used as the ground truth against which to train and validate the model. For example, an algorithm designed to interpret immunohistochemistry results on appropriately stained and scanned slides might use the pathologist interpretation as the ground truth and train the algorithm to replicate the pathologist's interpretation.[9] One downside of this approach is that the algorithm will never outperform the human when the human is treated as the gold standard.[10] In some tasks where there is substantial interhuman variability (eg, pathologist interpretation where different pathologists will disagree), a consensus among people can be used as the gold standard and then it is possible for the algorithm to outperform an individual person.[9] In cases where the algorithm is intended to perform tasks that are impossible for people to perform, verifiable endpoints other than direct human judgment are needed. For example, a pharmacogenomic algorithm that predicts individualized drug dosing based on patient genotypes might use clinical outcomes, blood drug concentrations or clinical responses[11] as an endpoint. In other cases, such as forecasting models, algorithms may be trained to predict some future state (eg, patient survival) based on currently available information.[8] Additional information on capturing ground truth targets is presented later (see question "How can ground truth targets be captured in the training and validation data?")

What are the Steps Involved in a Clinical Machine Learning Problem?

This topic is reviewed in greater detail in a prior Clinics in Laboratory Medicine article,[4] and the details will vary from problem to problem. A typical approach to the development of a clinical prediction model involves at least the following steps:

1. Problem conception and development
2. Data extraction, cleaning, and assembly
3. Model training
4. Model validation
5. Iteration on steps 1 to 4
6. Model implementation

Key aspects of these steps are described later in greater detail.

What is Involved in Problem Conception and Development?

This is often one of the most challenging aspects of the model development process and typically requires domain knowledge and human decision-making. One of the most important early steps is to define clear objectives. Although this sounds obvious, many projects start with high-level goals, for example, early detection of colon cancer. However, to develop a model, the investigator would need to be much more specific about which patients, in which settings, and with which predictors. Likewise, they would need to decide whether the goal is to detect early-stage tumors, late-stage tumors, or all tumors and how ground truth tumor status should be assessed. Often there are no right answers to these questions based on first principles, so likely the best approach is to consider the end application and work backward. Practical considerations such as data availability and ease of access may also come into play. Several specific decisions must be made as defined in **Table 1**.

Although there are many details that fall outside the scope of this table and article, once decisions listed in this table are made, a substantial portion of the cognitive work that goes into model development is complete.

How can Ground Truth Targets be Captured in the Training and Validation Data?

In general, supervised machine learning can be useful because it predicts attributes that would otherwise be difficult, impossible, or resource-intensive to assess. As a result, it is often challenging to capture ground truth prediction targets. Thus, sometimes creative framing is necessary to identify prediction tasks that are useful (it usually is not useful to predict something obvious) but also possible (it is not possible to train a model to predict something entirely unknowable). Some typical problem frameworks in the clinical space include the following:

- Using retrospective data to train a forecasting model: in this framework, ground truth target variable results are captured using what we know at present. However, predictions are made using only information that was available at some time in the past. For example, if we are developing a model to predict 1-year risk of

Table 1
Key decisions in framing a clinical machine learning project

Decision	What it is and what should be considered	Example Consider a Model to Predict a Patient's Risk of Myocardial Infarction Within 1 y	Area of Expertise
Inclusion criteria	Which patients or cases should we include in our training and validation? Which patients/settings? Generally, it should be designed to match the intended application	Patients 50 y or older presenting to their primary care doctor for a well visit	Clinical
Unit of analysis	The unit of analysis is what defines a "case" and generally what defines each unique row in the dataset. "Unique patients" is often the unit of analysis, but alternatives can include encounters and laboratory test collections, among many others. There will generally be one separate prediction made for each case as defined by the unit of analysis.	A primary care visit	Clinical
Target/outcome variable	The target variable is what we are trying to predict. This may in part be determined by the intended use, but practical considerations may also come into play to enable the target variable to be feasibly captured and programmatically defined. The target variable may be defined based on custom rules	New diagnosis of myocardial infarction as shown by either an ICD-10 code associated with acute myocardial infarction or an elevated troponin test result	Clinical

(continued on next page)

Decision	What it is and what should be considered	Example Consider a Model to Predict a Patient's Risk of Myocardial Infarction Within 1 y	Area of Expertise
Table 1 (*continued*)			
	incorporating multiple criteria. (eg, patient has a particular ICD code or is on a certain medication).		
Predictors	The predictors are the variables that the model will accept as inputs to predict the target. Similar to the target variable, both the intended application as well as practical considerations may come into play when selecting predictors. Domain expertise may help to identify predictors likely to be informative. Rule-based logic may be developed to "engineer" custom predictor variables based on a combination of underlying data elements.	• Results from lipid screening • # of first-degree relatives with heart disease • Systolic and diastolic blood pressure • Age • Gender • Smoking status • Diabetes • Key diagnoses	Clinical/Computational
Predictor representation	In many frameworks, this involves defining how predictors should be represented in the 2-dimensional table. For example, if a patient has multiple results for a given predictor variable, do we use the latest, the mean, the median, the range and so forth? Should a variable such as smoking status be captured as a single binary yes/no or should information about intensity of current and past use be	• Represent key diagnoses as multiple binary variables by applying a grouper to the patient problem list and encounter diagnoses over the prior 5 y. • Take the minimum, maximum, mean and count for blood pressure readings and laboratory test results	Clinical/Computational

	captured? Should diagnostic codes be grouped? If so, how? Over what time period?		
Approach to missing data	What should we do if a patient does not have a value for a predictor? For example, what if a laboratory test was not performed? This can be in part determined by practical factors such as the frequency of missing data but can also be informed by the end application. Often, imputation is used to predict the results of missing data elements based on available ones.	Random forest–based imputation as a possibility	Computational mostly (guided by clinician input)
Data sources	Where should we get the data? What systems or databases can be used?	Institutional enterprise data warehouse fed by the EHR systems	Clinical and clinical informatician
Number of cases	How many cases should be included in the training data? This is generally informed by model complexity. A more complex model requires more data.	1000 training; 100 parameter tuning; 100 validation	Computational
Model type and architecture	What type of model should we train? Often multiple model types are trained, and the best performing ones are ultimately used.	Random forest and logistic regression	Computational/clinical informatician to the extent it affects implementation
Performance metrics	What performance metrics should be used to evaluate the model? Generally, these should at minimum be applied to a randomly selected test partition of the data. It is sometimes ideal to demonstrate the performance of the model on a truly new dataset.	AUC, sensitivity, specificity, positive predictive value, negative predictive value	Clinical/computational

Abbreviation: EHR, electronic health record.

myocardial infarction, we might use data as of today to determine whether each patient had a myocardial infarction over the past year. We would then use as predictors only information that was available at least a year ago. In this way, we would apply the model to future patients using information currently available to predict the patient's myocardial infarction risk moving forward. Such approaches assume no inherent change over time; if for example, treatments aimed at preventing myocardial infarction had improved substantially since the training of our model, this type of approach may be invalid.

- Predicting the results of a costly, invasive, or resource-intensive diagnostic test: for example, we might train a model to predict the results of an invasive tissue biopsy using noninvasive laboratory markers. In this case, we might use patients who had the invasive biopsy for model training (with biopsy results serving as the ground truth target) but the model could nonetheless be useful to future patients if it helps them avoid biopsy.
- Use manual curation or the result of manual processes to develop models that seek to automate these processes: in this framework, we are attempting to automate or improve manual human tasks. For example, we might attempt to predict which medications a physician prescribes for a given patient. In this case, actual physician practice could serve as the ground truth, but the model could provide a foundation for clinical decision support for future patient encounters. This approach could be particularly useful if trained using highly specialized experts and then rolled out to less specialized clinicians. Similarly, algorithms may be trained to predict a pathologist's interpretation of a slide or a radiologist's interpretation of an image. Finally, in some cases, manual annotation may be performed for the purposes of model training. For example, a chart review could be used to identify anomalous laboratory test results and then a model could be trained to predict these.[20] Similarly, simulation can sometimes be used to generate cases with appropriate ground truth labels.[15]

What Does Data Extraction and Assembly Involve?

Many machine learning frameworks require the training and validation data to be structured as a 2-dimensional table with rows representing cases (eg, patients or whatever the unit of analysis is) and columns representing attributes of the case (predictor or target variables). Often, data are initially extracted from databases that compile data from underlying operational systems including in the clinical setting electronic health records (EHRs), low-intensity support services (LISs) and billing systems. In a typical framework, the data scientist or analyst must extract data from these databases and transform it into a 2-dimensional table. This process often involves considerable effort and must incorporate the framing decisions described in **Table 1**. For example, suppose we wish to build a model using predictors including the patients' mean glucose during their hospital admission with a unit of analysis of a "hospital admission." In this case, the underlying data might be in the form of a laboratory database with test results where each row represents a test result and information including the patient, collection time, test code, and result. To transform this into a 2-dimensional table for model training, we would need to extract from the laboratory database all relevant glucose results and then group them by patient-hospital-admission, taking the mean glucose per admission. Moreover, we would need to decide which glucose tests to include (eg, only main laboratory glucose results, point-of-care results, or both). Although not overly complex, this process, particularly when scaled across dozens or more predictors, can be quite time consuming. In practice, many data scientists spend a substantial portion of their time assembling and cleaning data.

Moreover, aggregating and formatting underlying data into a 2-dimensional table is only part of the process of data assembly. Most models require that the data be "clean," which might include among other things that no data elements are missing and that the values of predictor and outcome variables meet specific criteria. For example, if a glucose measurement is treated as a continuous variable, nonnumeric findings (eg, "<20 mg/dL") must be converted into a numeric form. Likewise, missing values may need to be addressed through processes including imputation. Categorical variables often require transformation through groupers or other frameworks; for example, most models will not be able to appropriately use all raw ICD10 diagnostic codes because there are far too many distinct codes (approximately 70,000 unique ICD10 codes). In such cases, it is often useful to group codes into related categories before feeding into the model.

Finally, a random sample of the data is often set aside for use in model validation. A common approach is to randomly sample a certain number of rows to hold out for use in testing. Twenty percent of the total cases are sometimes set aside for testing, but the specific percentage will vary. If the same patient is represented in multiple rows, which may happen if the unit of analysis is a patient encounter or something other than a patient, it would usually be appropriate to randomly sample patients to place into the training versus testing partition and not individual rows.

What Does Model Training Involve?

Once a clean dataset is assembled, the next step involves the model training. In many cases, this process is relatively straightforward. Commonly used programming languages including R[21] and Python[22] have a variety of open-source libraries that require only a few lines of code to train models using appropriately formatted training data. The simplicity to the end user often masks complex processes that are happening "under the hood."

The underlying training process will vary between model types, but, in general, model training involves optimizing model "parameters" to minimize a "cost" function. Parameters are coefficients, weights, logical rules, or other values that define how the model transforms inputs (predictors) into outputs (predictions of the target variable). The cost function determines how good the predictions are. Simple cost functions just compare the predictions to the ground truth values of the target. For example, a simple cost function for binary classification might just be the error rate (ie, proportion of training cases incorrectly classified, given a certain set of model parameters). Typical cost functions are more complex and may include "regularization" components to favor simpler models that will in turn be more likely to generalize. As described in more detail later in this article, regularized cost functions penalize a model both for incorrect predictions and complexity, such that the trained model will ideally balance 2 completing goals: prediction accuracy and model simplicity/ generalizability.

By way of example, consider a simple linear regression model to predict patients' hemoglobin A1c based on their age and body mass index (BMI). This model would have the following form:

$$\text{PredictedA1c}_{\text{patient}i} = W_0 + W_1 * \text{age}_{\text{patient}_i} + W_2 * \text{BMI}_{\text{patient}_1.}$$

In this case, the model has 3 parameters (W_0, W_1, W_2). The cost function might be the sum squared error as given:

$$Error = \sum_{all\ i} \left(PredictedA1c_{patient_i} - Actual\ A1c_{patient_1} \right)^2$$

The goal of training would then be to find the values of W_0, W_1, and W_2 that minimize this cost function. Of course, this model is likely to perform poorly, as age and BMI far from fully explain the variation in patient A1c values. We could imagine a more complex model that had additional weights (Ws) and additional predictors such as family history of diabetes, blood pressure, and prior A1c results. Such a model would likely perform better. However, if we select a model that has a large number of predictors relative to the size of the training data, the model will be prone to *overfitting* (see question "Why should model performance usually be assessed using held-out test data?").

One way to reduce the overfitting would be to use regularization. If regularization were to be used, the cost function might also include a penalty term that grows with the absolute value of each coefficient, besides the intercept term W_0, such that the model favors values of W that are closer to 0 unless increasing them would substantially improve the concordance between predicted and measured A1c. An intuitive way to think about regularization involves first considering the fact that adding an additional feature (predictor) to a model will generally add at least one additional coefficient, thereby increasing the freedom of the model to fit and the risk of overfitting (unregularized linear models will have an extra degree of freedom per predictor). Conversely, forcing the coefficient in front of a predictor to be 0 is the same as removing a predictor, thereby removing a degree of freedom from a linear model. Regularization strikes a balance between keeping and removing a predictor, by not forcing a coefficient to be 0 but by also not giving the model full range to fit the coefficient to any number from negative to positive infinity without an associated cost that must be overcome through improved performance.

In some cases, structural features of the model (known as hyperparameters) are also trained, a process often referred to as "hyperparameter tuning." Additional technical explanation of machine learning is provided in the article by McDermott and colleagues included in this issue.

What Does Model Validation Involve?

Model validation involves applying a trained machine learning model to held-out validation data to make predictions of the target variable. The predicted results are then compared with the actual results, and various performance metrics are computed. Although in some cases the performance metrics may parallel the cost function that was used in model training, these are often not the same. For example, regularization terms would generally not be factored into model performance metrics. (Because we are testing on held-out data, the performance measured in this step is usually taken as the generalizable model performance; thus there is no need to further reward predictions that were based on a simpler model).

In the case of classification models, common performance metrics include area under the receiver operating characteristic curve (AUroC), area under the precision-recall curve, F1, sensitivity, and specificity. Because AUroC only considers the relative values of predictions and the discriminative power of the model, probabilistic outputs should generally be assessed using a measure of calibration[23] (eg, Brier Loss) in addition to AUroC. For example, a sepsis model will achieve a high AUroC as long as the predicted probabilities for patients who do not have sepsis are lower than the predicted probabilities for patients who do. However, for the probabilities to be maximally meaningful, we would ideally like to see, for example, that approximately 1 in 10 patients with a predicted probability of sepsis actually do have sepsis. Likewise, if we apply the sepsis model to a population where 10% of patients have sepsis and the model outputs a 10% probability for every patient, the model will be well calibrated but would have no discriminative power and thus a poor AUroC. Thus, looking at AUroC and calibration together is usually important. In the case of regression models, mean squared error is sometimes used. Utilization of an external dataset separate from the one originally used for training and initial validation is ideal to demonstrate model generalizability.

Why Should Model Performance Usually be Assessed Using Held-Out Test Data?

A held-out set of test data (often generated as a random sample of the overall data as discussed earlier) is needed to assess generalizable model performance. In most cases, models will perform better if applied to their training data than on an independent set of test data; this is called overfitting and is almost inevitable to some degree. Overfitting happens because models will learn random nuances of the training data that do not generalize. Performance on held-out data not used in model training provides a better indicator of generalizable model performance on future cases after the model is applied in practice.

In some cases, a model is trained multiple times, using different training-testing splits; this can help in assessing sampling variation that might affect model performance. However, it is often best practice to set aside some data until the very end of the project. Only after the final model is trained and "locked down" are the set aside data used for validation. This way, the validation performance is most likely to capture the true generalizable performance of the model. If the validation data are considered during model development, the research may (often inadvertently) make decisions using the validation data that help improve validation performance. If this happens, the model may subtly learn nuances specific to the validation data, and thus the model performance on the validation data may not fully represent generalizable model performance.

What Form Does a Trained Model Take?

A trained model includes a structure/architecture and optimal parameter values established during training. Using as an example the hypothetical A1c regression model mentioned previously, the architecture/structure would be a linear regression model using age and BMI as predictors. The parameters would be the coefficients (W_0, W_1, W_2). More complex models such as deep learning models (described later) may include millions of parameters and complex architectures. Knowing the architecture and parameters would allow a suitably programmed computer to apply the model to future sets of predictors to make predictions.

What is Deep Learning?

This article thus far has mostly contemplated problems where the data can be represented in a structured form—usually a 2-dimensional table. Although this framework may work well for many types of clinical data—for example, laboratory test results can often be represented as cells in a table without undue effort—other types of data such as images (eg, radiology or anatomic pathology) or natural language (eg, unstructured clinical notes) are not easily represented in such formats. Many traditional attempts to apply machine learning to unstructured data such as images and text involves hand engineering features. For example, one might imagine trying to capture characteristics of a white blood cell viewed under a microscope such as cell size, shape, and nuclear to cytoplasmic ratio and then putting these values as features in a table. However, such approaches are often cumbersome to implement in practice because they require developing a hand-curated set of rules for each problem and extracting the information can remain difficult. For example, the researcher might need to code logic to enable the computer to identify the nucleus, the cytoplasm, and their respective sizes.

Modern advances in a subfield of machine learning, called "deep learning," allowed for the training of machine learning algorithms directly from unstructured data without needing to engineer features or represent the data in a structured form.[24] Deep learning generally involves complex neural networks that frequently include millions of parameters. Training deep learning models is often computationally intensive; however, specialized computer chips known as GPUs (graphical processing units) can facilitate training. Technical details of deep learning lie beyond the scope of this article but have been reviewed in depth in prior works.[25,26]

Deep learning has been applied to problems such as image classification (eg, identifying cancer in a whole slide image) and information extraction from natural language text (eg, determining whether a patient is a smoker based on a narrative clinical note). A class of deep learning models—known as generative models—can generate new synthetic data, for example, synthetic images that may be visually indistinguishable from real ones but that are generated by a computer.

What is Involved in Artificial Intelligence Model Deployment?

Successful training and validation of a machine learning model usually represents a critical project milestone and in some cases may represent the end goal. However, in most projects, model implementation is needed to achieve project goals. For example, a model intended to predict a patient's risk of sepsis may need to be implemented into clinical practice as a clinical decision support alert to achieve patient care benefits.

Depending on the model type, implementation may take many forms. For example, a sepsis prediction model might be most beneficial if implemented within the EHR to automatically provide decision support alerts in patients at high risk of sepsis. Although such a model might be feasible to deploy as an online calculator (requiring clinicians to manually input necessary patient data) or even a risk score intended for hand calculation, such approaches would usually be suboptimal. In particular, requiring a clinician to input results makes the model cumbersome and inconvenient for clinicians to use and may introduce manual data input errors. Moreover, such manually deployed models will only identify patients in whom the clinician already has sufficient suspicion of the underlying condition (eg, sepsis) to use the model.

Multianalyte assays with algorithmic analyses may be implemented within traditional LIS/EHR systems or within specialized interfaced platforms. Likewise, genomic algorithms may be integrated into the bioinformatics pipeline, and pathology image analysis algorithms may be integrated into the whole slide scanning processes including the image viewing software.

In practice, model implementation is complex and often represents one of the biggest barriers to greater adoption of clinical AI solutions.

Why is Model Implementation Challenging?

There are several key barriers to model implementation, including technical, administrative, evidential, and educational barriers. The technical barriers stem from the reality that many traditional health information systems (including EHR and LIS systems), although necessary for "last mile" delivery of decision support back to the clinician, are not well suited to implementation of AI models (see the article by Dighe later in this issue for additional information on EHR optimization to support machine learning.)

Although this situation is improving as EHR vendors expand their functionality, limitations remain. Some solutions rely on interfacing external decision support engines with the EHR, using Fast Healthcare Interoperability Resources[27,28] or other interfacing standards.

Perhaps more challenging than the technical details are the administrative ones. Regulatory requirements around clinical algorithms are often unclear (or at least perceived to be). Similarly, in practice, concerns around liability for algorithm errors are a common concern (regardless of the actual law, on which this investigator is not qualified to opine, clinicians, health systems, and vendors worry about legal liability created by following advice from decision support algorithms). Finally, institutional governance around EHR systems may be better equipped to address traditional types of clinical decisions than to address AI algorithms. Evidential barriers remain another challenge. Unlike some more traditional areas of laboratory medicine, the standards required to fully validate an algorithm's safety, efficacy, and clinical utility are ill-defined. Finally, as AI takes a greater role in health care, medical education will need to adapt to train clinicians in how best to interact with AI-based systems.

What is the Role of the Data Scientist and the Role of the Clinical Domain Expert?

In general, accomplishing the aforementioned steps requires multidisciplinary expertise, including clinical domain expertise, computational and machine learning expertise, and in most cases clinical informatics expertise. This clinical, computational, and informatics expertise can be supplied by multiple individuals; however, in the opinion of this investigator, it is often optimal if the individuals involved in the project have at least some cross-functional expertise as discussed later.

A typical project team might involve a clinician leader who can identify the clinical needs and frame the task involved (eg, specify decisions shown in **Table 2** tagged with "clinical"). It is likely useful for this person to have at least a basic knowledge of data science so that the project goals and tasks can be specified in a way that can be directly applied computationally. Likewise, understanding key concepts around data science will enable the clinician expert to better understand which tasks are "easier" and thus to frame the problem in a way that meets clinical goals while maximizing likelihood of success (or minimizing resources required to achieve success).

Likewise, a project team would generally involve a computational expert to opine on modeling frameworks, strategies for addressing missing data and other similar considerations (**Table 2**, rows tagged with "computational"). It is useful for this individual to have a working knowledge of the clinical considerations involved and especially limitations of clinical data to enable optimal decision-making. The computational expert in some cases might direct or advise a hands-on programmer or analyst (or trainee) who writes and executes the computer code necessary to carry out the analysis. Finally, expertise in clinical informatics is usually required to understand the underlying data sources, where to extract the data, and to understand the limitations. Clinical informatics expertise may similarly be necessary to advise on strategies for model implementation. In many cases, the clinical or computational expert will have sufficient informatics expertise to serve this role.

A key goal of this article is to provide individuals with clinical laboratory expertise a "study guide" to help them better serve as the clinical expert on clinical AI model development. Although knowledge beyond that contained herein would be optimal for an individual wishing to serve in this capacity, the investigator's hope is that this article can serve as a starting point. Although it is the investigator's opinion that individuals with extensive cross-functional expertise including the clinical, computational,

Table 2
Summarizes some potential applications of artificial intelligence in the laboratory

Category	Example
Image analysis	Determining whether a whole slide image contains cancer[12]
Diagnostic prediction	Predict the likelihood that a patient has sepsis[13]
Clinical forecasting	Predict a patient's likelihood of readmission within 30 d following hospital discharge[14]
Detection of preanalytic errors	Identification of wrong blood in tube errors[15]
Test result prediction	Predict ferritin test results[16]
Analyze human-EHR interaction/EHR optimization	Predict the likelihood that a clinician will accept a clinical decision support alert[17]
Natural language processing	Extract patient diagnoses and attributes from free text notes[18]
Multianalyte assays with algorithmic analysis	Noninvasive assessment of liver fibrosis using serum biomarkers[19]
Genotypic analysis	Predict whether a genomic variant of uncertain significance explains a patient's phenotype (see article by Danielle Kurant later in this issue for additional information)

Abbreviation: EHR, electronic health record.

and informatics aspects of the project are optimally suited to solving certain challenges in the clinical AI space, many problems can be solved very effectively by multidisciplinary teams, and formation of such team is highly encouraged.

DISCUSSION

Although medicine is behind many other industries in terms of development and adoption of AI-based systems, general approaches developed outside of health care are likely to increasingly offer opportunities to improve the efficiency, precision, and efficacy of laboratory diagnostics and clinical care. Nonetheless, as summarized in this article, nuances of health care data, systems, and infrastructure create barriers to wider adoption. As more pathologists, clinicians, and laboratorians gain a better understanding of laboratory AI and the current barriers and opportunities, we as a field may begin to better conquer these challenges and deploy AI toward higher quality care and better patient outcomes.

DISCLOSURE

J. Baron is an employee of Roche Diagnostics and has equity in Roche as part of his employee compensation. This article was prepared within his academic capacity and in no way in the context of his role at Roche.

REFERENCES

1. Baron JM, Dighe AS. Computerized provider order entry in the clinical laboratory. J Pathol Inform 2011;2:35 [published Online First: Epub Date].

2. Baron JM, Dighe AS, Arnaout R, et al. The 2013 symposium on pathology data integration and clinical decision support and the current state of field. J Pathol Inform 2014;5:2 [published Online First: Epub Date].

3. Baron JM, Dighe AS. The role of informatics and decision support in utilization management. Clin Chim Acta 2014;427:196–201 [published Online First: Epub Date].

4. Baron JM, Kurant DE, Dighe AS. Machine learning and other emerging decision support tools. Clin Lab Med 2019;39(2):319–31 [published Online First: Epub Date]|.

5. Louis DN, Feldman M, Carter AB, et al. Computational pathology. Arch Pathol Lab Med 2015. https://doi.org/10.5858/arpa.2015-0093-SA [published Online First: Epub Date]|.

6. Louis DN, Gerber GK, Baron JM, et al. Computational pathology: an emerging definition. Arch Pathol Lab Med 2014;138(9):1133–8 [published Online First: Epub Date]|.

7. Lee LH, Mansoor A, Wood B, et al. Performance of CellaVision DM96 in leukocyte classification. J Pathol Inform 2013;4:14 [published Online First: Epub Date]|.

8. Baron JM, Paranjape K, Love T, et al. Development of a "meta-model" to address missing data, predict patient-specific cancer survival and provide a foundation for clinical decision support. J Am Med Inform Assoc 2021;28(3):605–15 [published Online First: Epub Date]|.

9. Ibrahim A, Gamble P, Jaroensri R, et al. Artificial intelligence in digital breast pathology: techniques and applications. Breast 2020;49:267–73 [published Online First: Epub Date]|.

10. Jahn SW, Plass M, Moinfar F. Digital pathology: advantages, limitations and emerging perspectives. J Clin Med 2020;9(11) [published Online First: Epub Date]|.

11. Lin E, Lin CH, Lane HY. Machine learning and deep learning for the pharmacogenomics of antidepressant treatments. Clin Psychopharmacol Neurosci 2021;19(4):577–88 [published Online First: Epub Date]|.

12. Dimitriou N, Arandjelovic O, Caie PD. Deep learning for whole slide image analysis: an overview. Front Med (Lausanne) 2019;6:264 [published Online First: Epub Date]|.

13. Fleuren LM, Klausch TLT, Zwager CL, et al. Machine learning for the prediction of sepsis: a systematic review and meta-analysis of diagnostic test accuracy. Intensive Care Med 2020;46(3):383–400 [published Online First: Epub Date]|.

14. Krittanawong C, Zhang H, Wang Z, et al. Artificial intelligence in precision cardiovascular medicine. J Am Coll Cardiol 2017;69(21):2657–64 [published Online First: Epub Date]|.

15. Rosenbaum MW, Baron JM. Using machine learning-based multianalyte delta checks to detect wrong blood in tube errors. Am J Clin Pathol 2018;150(6):555–66 [published Online First: Epub Date]|.

16. Luo Y, Szolovits P, Dighe AS, et al. Using machine learning to predict laboratory test results. Am J Clin Pathol 2016;145(6):778–88 [published Online First: Epub Date]|.

17. Baron JM, Huang R, McEvoy D, et al. Use of machine learning to predict clinical decision support compliance, reduce alert burden, and evaluate duplicate laboratory test ordering alerts. JAMIA Open 2021;4(1):ooab006 [published Online First: Epub Date]|.

18. Zeng Z, Deng Y, Li X, et al. natural language processing for EHR-based computational phenotyping. Ieee/acm Trans Comput Biol Bioinform 2019;16(1):139–53 [published Online First: Epub Date]|.
19. Chou R, Wasson N. Blood tests to diagnose fibrosis or cirrhosis in patients with chronic hepatitis C virus infection: a systematic review. Ann Intern Med 2013; 158(11):807–20 [published Online First: Epub Date]|.
20. Baron JM, Mermel CH, Lewandrowski KB, et al. Detection of preanalytic laboratory testing errors using a statistically guided protocol. Am J Clin Pathol 2012; 138(3):406–13 [published Online First: Epub Date].
21. R Core Team. R: A Language and Environment for Statistical Computing, 2013. Available at: https://cran.microsoft.com/snapshot/2014-09-08/web/packages/dplR/vignettes/xdate-dplR.pdf.
22. Pedregosa F, Varoquaux G, Gramfort A, et al. Scikit-learn: machine learning in Python. J machine Learn Res 2011;12:2825–30.
23. Bates DW, Auerbach A, Schulam P, et al. Reporting and implementing interventions involving machine learning and artificial intelligence. Ann Intern Med 2020; 172(11 Suppl):S137–44 [published Online First: Epub Date]|.
24. McBee MP, Awan OA, Colucci AT, et al. Deep learning in radiology. Acad Radiol 2018;25(11):1472–80 [published Online First: Epub Date]|.
25. Esteva A, Robicquet A, Ramsundar B, et al. A guide to deep learning in healthcare. Nat Med 2019;25(1):24–9, published Online First: Epub Date]|.
26. Miotto R, Wang F, Wang S, et al. Deep learning for healthcare: review, opportunities and challenges. Brief Bioinform 2018;19(6):1236–46 [published Online First: Epub Date]|.
27. Boussadi A, Zapletal E. A fast healthcare interoperability resources (FHIR) layer implemented over i2b2. BMC Med Inform Decis Mak 2017;17(1):120 [published Online First: Epub Date]|.
28. Mandel JC, Kreda DA, Mandl KD, et al. SMART on FHIR: a standards-based, interoperable apps platform for electronic health records. J Am Med Inform Assoc 2016;23(5):899–908 [published Online First: Epub Date]|.

Electronic Health Record Optimization for Artificial Intelligence

Anand S. Dighe, MD, PhD

KEYWORDS

- Clinical decision support • Electronic health record • Artificial intelligence
- Clinical laboratory

KEY POINTS

- Most artificial intelligence algorithms rely on predictors and outcomes that are structured. The lack of standards and low data quality can limit the direct use of EHR data in algorithm development.
- Standardization and harmonization of EHR dictionaries are a foundational step in creating a sustainable laboratory CDS program.
- The development of standardized approaches to extract data from the EHR, including FHIR and OpenCDS, may enable direct use of EHR data for CDS, but only if attention is paid to data quality and structure.

INTRODUCTION

The electronic health record (EHR) has become an increasingly important part of the way that clinical care is delivered. The types and density of data collected and stored in the EHR have increased to the point where nearly the entirety of a patient's health history may be present in the EHR. However, despite the high data content, much of the EHR clinical data are challenging to use directly in artificial intelligence (AI) algorithms because of a lack of standardization.[1] The reuse of EHR data for secondary purposes is typically time and resource intensive in part because of the need to analyze and validate EHR data before its use in decision support algorithms.[2] There have been recent studies demonstrating applications of secondary use of EHR data to predict outcomes that do not rely on harmonized or standardized EHR data, although it remains to be seen if these strategies can be used accurately and safely in clinical practice.[3–5]

The EHR provides numerous opportunities to provide laboratory-focused clinical decision support (CDS), including AI-based approaches.[6] However, most applications of

Department of Pathology, Massachusetts General Hospital, Harvard Medical School, 55 Fruit Street, Boston, MA 02114-2696, USA
E-mail address: asdighe@partners.org

Clin Lab Med 43 (2023) 17–28
https://doi.org/10.1016/j.cll.2022.09.003
0272-2712/23/© 2022 Elsevier Inc. All rights reserved.

AI require the predictor variables to be structured. Although laboratory test results would seem to be inherently structured and therefore directly suitable for use, in practice there are numerous areas of the laboratory order and results build that require careful attention during build and maintenance to support CDS efforts.[7] Furthermore, the ability to deliver effective decision support necessitates not only attention to the EHR build, but also an infrastructure that supports monitoring, testing, and knowledge discovery.

EHR semantic interoperability is the ability of an EHR to provide another system, whether another EHR or an internal or external CDS algorithm, with data having an unambiguous, shared meaning.[8,9] From the standpoint of clinical predictive model development, a common consideration is whether two data elements (eg, results from two laboratory tests sharing the same name in the EHR but produced in different laboratories) are equivalent and can be treated as a single feature in the model. Likewise, models may include variables or structural features to account for related but not identical data elements. For example, in some models, it may be appropriate to include laboratory results from the same analyte measured using different analytic methods as a single feature but to also include a second variable in the model denoting the source of the test result; this way model might learn any differences between the methods that are relevant to the outcome of interest. However, such modeling is only feasible if the underlying data are properly structured and captured in association with key metadata.

The realization of semantic interoperability requires structuring of the underlying data and structuring of the messaging format. In terms of the messaging format, HL7 fast health care information resources (FHIR) has emerged as a de facto standard for the interchange of clinical information. EHR vendors and health care providers have developed transformations between EHRs and the corresponding FHIR representations. However, structuring the underlying data remains a challenge for EHRs, despite the widespread availability of standardized approaches to represent EHR data.[10]

In this article we review the types of EHR data that are the basis of key aspects of laboratory CDS and potential AI algorithms. In addition to laboratory results, fundamental data in the EHR particularly relevant to laboratory CDS includes diagnosis, demographics, medical history, medications, and procedures. Because of the central role of laboratory testing in the diagnostic process, in this article we include a particular focus on the EHR data representing test orders, results, and diagnosis. We discuss the current state of standardization and the techniques for the extraction and use of laboratory and diagnosis data for AI-based CDS.

LABORATORY RESULT IDENTIFICATION

A key component of laboratory-based AI is the prerequisite to identify several fundamental aspects of each laboratory result. Logical Observation Identifiers Names and Codes (LOINC) is a database and universal standard that provides standardized tests names and codes for laboratory observations.[11,12] Each LOINC record corresponds to a single test or group of tests (ie, test panel). LOINC specifies the name, property measured, timing, sample type, units of measure, and method (where relevant). In the United States, LOINC has been a part of most EHR laboratory observations because of governmental incentives for the use of LOINC during the exchange of laboratory data. When laboratories and health systems implement LOINC, the LOINC code (eg, 2160–0, for plasma creatinine) chosen by the laboratory needs to be carefully selected by a team that has knowledge of the functionality and limitations of LOINC. The current version of LOINC has more than 80,000 clinical observation and laboratory codes. The selection process of a given LOINC code from the LOINC database of codes is not a standardized process and typically individual laboratories assign LOINC codes based on their local process. More recently, laboratory instrument and reagent vendors have begun to include LOINC recommendations in their package inserts to assist laboratories with this task. Newly developed laboratory assays may not have a LOINC code defined at the time of the initial test launch. Several studies have examined LOINC code assignments in different institutions and the variability in LOINC for identical tests is such that the variation would be expected to create interoperability challenges for analytics.[13,14] In addition to selection of the appropriate LOINC code, the units of measure for a given result need to be machine readable for optimal use of the results in analytic engines. The Unified Code for Units of Measure (UCUM) provides a syntax and system to express and convert between all common units encountered in a laboratory setting.[15] Another similar terminology system similar to LOINC, the Nomenclature for Properties and Units (NPU), is used predominantly in northern Europe.

Many CDS and AI algorithms rely on individual test result values to be categorized and stored in the EHR as "normal" or "abnormal" or "high" or "low" to be able to be used in decision support algorithms without additional processing. For many laboratory tests, the numeric value of the result may not hold much meaning for an analytic without the provision of a result flag to provide a structured understanding whether the reported value is low, normal, or high compared with a healthy population. Result flagging is also clinically important in EHR displays, highlighting abnormal results to ensure that results are recognized, and appropriate action taken, and allowing triage of these results during clinical work-ups. For quantitative results, flags on test results can be configured to describe the degree of abnormality (eg, a different value for high, low, critical high, critical low, or a change from prior value). Although the flags associated with a numeric result may be helpful for a given analytic, the application of flags is not standardized and there is high variability between laboratories regarding what result values are flagged and how results are flagged.[16]

For qualitative results, such as microbiology testing, flags are often set at the finding level, with likely pathogenic organisms generating "abnormal" or "critical abnormal" flagging.

In addition to using LOINC, microbiology culture results are supported by specific SNOMED-CT concept hierarchies for organism, clinical findings, and substance. The organism's name, resistance pattern, and antibiotic names can all be mapped to SNOMED-CT codes that enable standardized reporting and secondary use of these results.[17] Some systems, particularly anatomic pathology systems, have a limited ability to flag results as abnormal. Results generated from these systems (eg, Pap smears, biopsies) thus may be at risk of being overlooked clinically and may be challenging to incorporate into AI algorithms. In these instances, alternative approaches for clinically applying flags to abnormal results in the EHR may be needed, including interface engine programming to evaluate result values and apply flags to result messages before posting in the EHR. For use in AI and CDS, various postprocessing steps, such as using natural language processing, may be applied, but these technologies may introduce an unacceptable amount of noise or error.[18] Data extraction and normalization challenges are compounded when pooling data across multiple sources, such as from different institutions. The recommended approach is to have the source system (eg, the laboratory information system [LIS]) apply and send the flag to the EHR in a format that can readily be understood by the EHR for clinical display and storage with the result.

Another challenge using flagged results in AI algorithms are results generated outside the primary LIS, including outside reference laboratories or directly interfaced results that bypass the LIS and are reported directly into the EHR. Interfaces from such laboratories may not send flags or may send them in a different format that needs custom mapping to the EHR. These interfaced results may present significant blind spots for AI algorithms because these unflagged results may be treated as normal or even bypassed completely.

Moreover, there are several entire categories of test results that are challenging to incorporate into the EHR, and these results may remain unavailable for laboratory result-based analytics. These include point-of-care results, externally entered results, and historical results converted from other EHRs. Unless these result types are entered or transmitted in a structured, standardized format they will be inaccessible to many provider workflows and CDS tools within the EHR, and external analytics will be unable to use these results. A related challenge is the handling of results from external EHRs that are capable of sharing data with the primary EHR. EHR vendors are increasingly enabling the sharing of laboratory data between institutions, most recently through FHIR interfaces. With this functionality, EHRs can accept and file results natively to the primary EHR database. Although potentially of high value, this technology presents challenges and risks. Given the differences between methods, flagging, reference ranges, and result interpretation between institutions, significant analysis needs to be done to decide whether to allow external laboratory data to populate CDS algorithms. Standardized nomenclatures, such as LOINC, may be useful in mapping results between institutions. However, given the variation between organizational LOINC implementations, it remains to be seen whether this is a practical means of automatically matching results without the time-intensive analysis of the LOINC codes used along with review of a representative selection of the incoming results.[12] Although EHR vendors provide tools for mapping results, a detailed comparison at the level of individual orders and results may be necessary to ensure the quality and safety of result mappings.

LABORATORY INTERPRETIVE COMMENTS

In addition to the result values provided, interpretive comments are a critical part of many laboratory reports.[19] One type of interpretive comment is authored by an expert pathologist/laboratorian to provide a summary of a panel of individual result measurements and put these results in the context of the patient's current clinical state.[20,21] For example, hypercoagulation laboratory work-ups may be accompanied by a text-based pathologist interpretation that summarizes the findings and provide recommendations for diagnosis and treatment. These interpretive comments are of critical importance for the accurate interpretation of the testing because they may call attention to likely interferences or preanalytic influences. The second important class of interpretive comments are those that may be automatically appended to the result by a calculation within the LIS. These sorts of comments may indicate the presence of factors, such as hemolysis, lipemia, lack of fasting, or other variables that could affect the accuracy of the measurement or interpretation. Analytics generally fail to incorporate either of these types of interpretive comments into their algorithms and this can impact the reliability of such algorithms. Ongoing efforts to improve the quality, standardization, and harmonization of interpretive comments may result in the future ability to integrate these key laboratory report elements into analytics.[22,23]

LABORATORY NAMES FOR ELECTRONIC HEALTH RECORD–BASED CLINICAL DECISION SUPPORT

Although LOINC provides a standardized approach to extract and exchange data between systems, laboratory result naming within the EHR itself typically uses an internal cataloging of result components to classify similar result components as having a "common name" reflecting observations sharing the same name, units of measure, and similar result value characteristics.[7] Although LOINC does provide a system for test names including a short name, display name, and consumer name, these may or may not have traction with clinicians and often historical names may be used for orders and results. For example the LOINC display name of "F5 gene targeted mutation analysis" would be confusing to many providers who may be more familiar with the historic name of factor V Leiden mutation polymerase chain reaction. This locally curated common name is often the basis for the way laboratories studies are displayed in EHR grids or flowsheets to permit providers to more easily review related test results and view trends in test results over time. Although these naming approaches are important to allow clinical integration of test results, the accuracy and robustness of decision support rules and algorithms implemented within the EHR may be highly dependent on the locally designated common names of the various result components. Furthermore, because external CDS and AI efforts often rely on reports or extracts from the EHR based on these common names, the fidelity and accuracy of analytics can also suffer when these mappings are missing or inaccurate. In addition to their unavailability for AI, mismapped or unmapped results may be at increased risk of being missed by providers when reviewing laboratory results. A related issue can occur when multicomponent results (eg, a hypercoagulation panel containing many individual tests) are not reported in a single report, creating a situation where the individual positive or negative result components may be reported separately from one another, complicating interpretation, especially by analytics. The use of EHR reports and related auditing tools to periodically monitor systems for unmapped or mismapped test results is recommended.

INTERHOSPITAL STANDARDIZATION

Many health care organizations consist of a network of sites. In cases where these organizations have grown by merger and acquisition, there may exist multiple clinical laboratories with different instruments and possibly different information systems (LIS and/or EHR). In these settings the interoperability of laboratory orders and results is a significant concern and has implications for the CDS in this environment. Harmonization is the process of standardizing orders, results, reports, and result interpretation criteria. This process is a challenging and time-consuming undertaking, requiring strong central governance and long-term commitment. Nonharmonized systems face several CDS challenges. For numerous clinical EHR workflows logic must be built and maintained to account for the variation in codes and result interpretation between sites. When possible, systems should harmonize the laboratory build, including order and result codes, reference ranges, flagging, critical values and reflex protocols between the sites within the organization. The interoperability of laboratory data is necessary to lower build complexity and facilitate internal and external analytic approaches.

MOLECULAR RESULTS

Despite rapid progress in the understanding of the genetic basis of many diseases, genetic information in the EHR is sparse and at least in the case of genome-wide studies and large multigene panels, results are rarely structured in formats usable for AI and CDS. The EHR has been largely designed and optimized to access and display the most recent diagnostic testing with transient value, whereas genetic testing, which may have lifelong implications for the patient, is challenging to access and extract for decision support purposes.[24] Unlike more common laboratory tests, results from genomic and complex genetic tests are typically free text with no set result structure, no result flagging, and additionally results may be reported in formats, such as PDF, that are not amenable to extraction and reporting. Furthermore, a molecular diagnostic report is considered to have several layers, including the text interpretation provided to clinicians, the known genetic variants identified, and the raw sequencing data. In most cases, only the top layer, the text interpretation of the results, is available in the EHR. The standardization of genetic variant reporting and the storage of this information in the EHR in a standardized, retrievable form is necessary before genetic information can be readily included in AI algorithms. Recently several molecular reporting ontologies have started to become de facto standards including LOINC (for naming of orders and results), and such systems as International System for Human Cytogenetic Nomenclature (for cytogenetics) and Human Genome Variation Society nomenclature (for sequence variants). EHR developers are starting to incorporate genomic and genetic information to allow these data to be filed, stored, and displayed within the EHR. The ability to store germline and somatic variants in a standardized format within the EHR allows genomic variant–based alerting and reporting based on genomic variant data. Furthermore, FHIR protocols that can make use of the developing genomic standards are in development that promise the ability to extract and transmit genetic and genomic information between systems.[25]

ANATOMIC PATHOLOGY REPORTING

It has been long recognized that the content and structure of anatomic pathology reports play a major role in ensuring quality patient management.[26,27] The use of synoptic anatomic pathology checklist reports and attention to report formatting to optimize clinical utility have been demonstrated to be key facets of a quality system. However, these approaches alone, unless paired with mapping of the synoptic elements to a standardized vocabulary, do not make pathology data suitable for analytics. The goal of fully "computable" pathology reports is challenging because of the insufficient concept definitions in SNOMED-CT and LOINC for defining all the elements of the order and result.[28,29] In addition to having this mapping stored in the LIS it is important to have these mappings available in the EHR to facilitate decision support, data sharing, and reporting.

FAST HEALTH CARE INTEROPERABILITY RESOURCES AND OPEN CLINICAL DECISION SUPPORT

The HL7 FHIR is a standard for health care information exchange that is supported by most EHR vendors.[30] It permits data to be extracted from the EHR by systems without requiring the system to have knowledge of how the data are stored in the EHR. The use of FHIR to retrieve laboratory data requires knowledge of the LOINC codes used for a particular observation to store the data in the EHR. Because of the existence of many LOINC codes for highly related concepts, it is imperative that applications reliant on FHIR for laboratory data have knowledge of the diversity of LOINC codes that may be used by a given site's EHR to represent laboratory testing. For example, for a common analyte, such as blood creatinine, there are numerous LOINC codes that an EHR could use for a given result, depending on the clinical scenario (eg, timed or not, predialysis), units of measure, and specimen type. Lack of knowledge of the local LOINC code usage for the test can render critical laboratory data invisible to FHIR-based analytics.

OpenCDS is a collaborative effort to develop open-source, standards-based CDS tools.[31] The tools of OpenCDS, including CDS Hooks, permit software external to the EHR to access relevant EHR patient data and then return decision support back to the clinician within the standard workflow of a given EHR. The "hook" in CDS Hooks is a specific point within the EHR workflow with contextual information that is provided as part of the request to the CDS service. Each CDS service requires specific FHIR resources to provide the decision support that the EHR requests. OpenCDS is highly dependent on the underlying codification of the data because without semantic inter-operability the query does not return the requested data.

DATA IMPUTATION

Perhaps the biggest challenges to analyzing clinical data are data accuracy, completeness, and heterogeneity. Real-world data never include every data element that might be potentially useful for a given AI model. Laboratory testing is generally performed only episodically, so at any given time few patients will have values for all the laboratory tests that would be useful for a given algorithm. Traditional machine learning models work best (or only work for some machine learning algorithms) with datasets that contain a value for every predictor. Constructing a complete clinical dataset is often impossible and can limit algorithm use to only a small subset of patients that have all the predictor variables, reducing utility and introducing bias.[32] Many laboratory-based AI algorithms are developed using training sets that have a rich collection of results, often in patients receiving high-intensity inpatient care. In practice, however, patients have widely varying levels of laboratory testing and often do not have recent values for key analytes of importance for the developed algorithm. This can particularly be true if the algorithm relies on analytes in a narrow time range. Imputation is a potential solution for the issue of missing data. In imputation, the missing data are filled in using a variety of techniques including nearest neighbor analysis and multivariate imputation.[33] Imputation can compensate for the sparse laboratory data that is common in a medical record. Well-designed imputation can enable predictions to occur even in situations where many of the predictor variables may be outside the time window of a traditional algorithm.[34]

DIAGNOSIS CODING

Because laboratory testing–based algorithms are frequently designed to diagnose or rule out disease, it is readily apparent that the diagnosis-related information in the EHR would be valuable for laboratory-focused algorithms. However, there are several challenges because of the variety of ways that diagnostic information is stored and the standards available for diagnostic data. There are many categories of "diagnoses" in a given patient's EHR. These categories include problem lists (ambulatory and hospital), encounter diagnoses, admitting diagnoses, discharge diagnoses, patient medical/surgical history, and billing diagnoses.[35] Although many of these diagnoses are mapped to standards, including International Classification of Diseases, 10th edition (ICD-10), Common Procedural Terminology (CPT), Diagnosis-Related Group (DRG), and SNOMED-CT, there remains a challenge to holistically use the diagnostic information of the EHR. One challenge of these controlled vocabularies is inherent to EHR documentation in general, namely the cost versus perceived benefit by those entering the data (clinicians) and those who later analyze it (researchers and data scientists). Clinicians have little incentive to select the most accurate code or even to document the diagnosis in standardized formats or locations. Doing so typically takes additional time, something increasingly busy providers conserve for taking care of individual patients. For example, ICD-10 has more than 150,000 different diagnostic codes with overlaid rules that determine which code is appropriate for a given context. For ICD-10, payors often require the most specific of many similar codes for billing purposes. The challenge for each EHR is to map clinical documentation to these classification systems in an accurate fashion. In addition, there is no requirement that a given clinical document be tied to ICD-10 versus SNOMED-CT. ICD-10 and SNOMED-CT do not directly map to one another and crosswalks between these classifications are suboptimal, with the migration paths between classifications incomplete.[36] One such system, the Unified Medical Language System, was designed to integrate the abundance of standards and document the relationships between similar terms in different standards.[37] The Unified Medical Language System integrates more than 50 different source standards and aims to define the semantic relationships between standards and provide tools for the natural language processing of results.

Because of the wide variety of diagnostic data in the EHR, many CDS and AI algorithms rely primarily on a single source of diagnostic information (eg, problem lists). This is an error-prone approach because there is significant heterogeneity in the completeness of any diagnostic source, such as the problem list between institutions. When analyzed, success factors for problem list completeness at a given organization included financial incentives, use of problem-based charting, direct linkages to billing codes, and organizational culture.[38] However, studies that have combined diagnoses from multiple locations within the EHR (eg, encounter diagnosis, billing codes, problem lists, and medical history) have reported higher levels of accuracy and in some studies combinatorial approaches have exceeded the performance of manual record review.[39] The challenge of combining these data sources in an automated, accurate way that enables the combined diagnostic signal to be used for analytics remains a key goal for decision support to be able to incorporate this key EHR information. One method of aggregating and integrating diagnostic information for a particular patient involves the use of an EHR registry. Manually created registries have long been used to identify cohorts with various conditions (eg, diabetes, asthma) to be able to monitor the health of these populations via reporting and decision support.[40,41] EHR systems can permit the automatic creation of registries based on defining inclusion criteria for a given condition. For example, an EHR registry for diabetes could add patients to the diabetes registry that have a diagnosis of diabetes on their problem list, encounter diagnosis, billing diagnosis, or have an elevated hemoglobin A_{1c} test result. The ability to provide this registry information to CDS and AI algorithms can permit disparate and inconsistently documented diagnostic information to still support a CDS and AI program.

DATA PROVENANCE

Provenance is the provision of source information about a given piece of data that can supply key insights into the validity and quality of the data and how useful it may be for analytics.[42] For laboratory testing key metadata that may be important can include the reporting laboratory, the particular analyzer the testing is performed on, and the method of data entry (eg, interfaced or manually entered). Similarly with diagnosis data the source of the data (eg, entry by the provider, scheduling staff, billing office, reflex algorithm) and the timing of the information (preprocedure, discharge diagnosis) can provide useful information regarding the likely accuracy of the information. Algorithm developers may develop rules to exclude certain data elements believed to be unreliable based on their source. Moreover, sophisticated algorithms may learn to place different emphasis on superficially similar elements of data depending on the

Data Element	Standards	Challenges
Table 1		
Challenges for analytic use of laboratory-related data		
Test observation name/code	LOINC, CPT, NPU	Inconsistent and nonstandardized use of LOINC codes Lack of processes at sites to identify mismapped or unmapped results Lack of LOINC codes for newer test results
Test result units	UCUM, LOINC, NPU	Standardized units not reported by all laboratories Results with identical numeric values may be reported using different units (mg/L and μg/mL)
Specimen sources	SNOMED-CT	SNOMED-CT may not be sufficiently descriptive to handle all possible sources Use of unmapped "other" and free text sources
Test interpretive comments	None	"Atomic" results for a diagnostic work-up may not include the free text interpretation that may be generated for the evaluation (eg, hypercoagulation work-up with pathologist evaluation) Highly informative free text interpretations may be essentially invisible to analytics unless mapped (eg, to SNOMED-CT) Key comments that may invalidate or create uncertainly about the result (eg, presence of hemolysis, clotting) are largely free text and may not be available to the analytic
Diagnosis	ICD-10, SNOMED-CT, DRG	Inconsistent location for diagnosis documentation in EHR (problem list, encounter diagnosis, billing diagnosis) Diagnosis coding not a priority task for clinical workflows so accuracy is inconsistent Context for diagnosis important but inconsistently provided to analytics Lack of tools to aggregate and normalize disparate diagnostic information

source and its corresponding reliability. When provenance data are not available to the algorithms, model performance may suffer because "noisy" data are used in training or application and unreliable data may cause clinically important errors.

MAPPING AND MONITORING

The laboratory build for order and result components is the essential foundation for laboratory-based CDS and AI. Any components that are not mapped (or are not accurately mapped) to standardized vocabulary (eg, LOINC) are essentially invisible to CDS and analytics. Manual approaches to this mapping are resource- and time-intensive. In addition, mapping is not a one-time task, because the laboratory build is constantly evolving, with changes in test menus, build optimization, new acquisitions, and the introduction of new terms to the mapping vocabularies all introducing change to the system. Approaches to mapping must not only provide environments for comparison and mapping of terms but must also be capable of continuous monitoring for changes in the build and the introduction of unmapped or obsolete mappings. Software tools are starting to become available from EHR vendors and independent groups that permit rapid cycle build comparison to assist and normalize the process of term mapping.[43] Breakdowns in system-to-system interfaces may impact patient care and CDS. In addition, individual issues are often challenging to detect. For example, the failure of the single test to be filed properly in the EHR database because of an interface mapping issue may not be readily observed and could persist for long periods of time. Periodic system monitoring and audits are required to identify and address these latent errors before they impact CDS and AI algorithms.

SUMMARY

In this article we have reviewed the state of laboratory-related EHR data and its suitability for use in CDS and AI algorithms (**Table 1**). We also addressed the underlying harmonization and infrastructure required to scale and stabilize the laboratory build across an enterprise health care environment. The laboratory build should not only be focused on workflow and clinical review, but should be thoughtfully designed, implemented, and monitored such that the by-product of EHR laboratory workflows is a rich and standardized source of data that can be used internally and externally for AI-based algorithms with minimal preanalytic processing.

REFERENCES

1. Milinovich A, Kattan MW. Extracting and utilizing electronic health data from Epic for research. Ann Transl Med 2018;6(3):42.
2. Fort D, Weng C, Bakken S, et al. Considerations for using research data to verify clinical data accuracy. AMIA Jt Summits Transl Sci Proc 2014;2014:211–7.
3. Rajkomar A, Oren E, Chen K, et al. Scalable and accurate deep learning with electronic health records. NPJ Digit Med 2018;1:18.
4. Miotto R, Li L, Kidd BA, et al. Deep patient: an unsupervised representation to predict the future of patients from the electronic health records. Sci Rep 2016; 6:26094.
5. Lippi G. Machine learning in laboratory diagnostics: valuable resources or a big hoax? Diagnosis (Berl) 2019;8(2):133–5.
6. Baron JM, Kurant DE, Dighe AS. Machine learning and other emerging decision support tools. Clin Lab Med 2019;39(2):319–31.
7. Rudolf JW, Dighe AS. Decision support tools within the electronic health record. Clin Lab Med 2019;39(2):197–213.
8. de Mello BH, Rigo SJ, da Costa CA, et al. Semantic interoperability in health records standards: a systematic literature review. Health Technol (Berl) 2022;12(2): 255–72.

9. Moreno-Conde A, Moner D, Cruz WD, et al. Clinical information modeling processes for semantic interoperability of electronic health records: systematic review and inductive analysis. J Am Med Inform Assoc 2015;22(4):925–34.

10. Ferrão JC, Oliveira MD, Janela F, et al. Preprocessing structured clinical data for predictive modeling and decision support. A roadmap to tackle the challenges. Appl Clin Inform 2016;7(4):1135–53.

11. Uchegbu C, Jing X. The potential adoption benefits and challenges of LOINC codes in a laboratory department: a case study. Health Inf Sci Syst 2017;5(1):6.

12. Stram M, Gigliotti T, Hartman D, et al. Logical Observation Identifier Names and Codes for laboratorians. Arch Pathol Lab Med 2020;144(2):229–39.

13. Baorto DM, Cimino JJ, Parvin CA, et al. Using Logical Observation Identifier Names and Codes (LOINC) to exchange laboratory data among three academic hospitals. Proc AMIA Annu Fall Symp 1997;96–100.

14. Lin MC, Vreeman DJ, McDonald CJ, et al. Correctness of voluntary LOINC mapping for laboratory tests in three large institutions. AMIA Annu Symp Proc 2010;2010:447–51.

15. Schadow G, McDonald CJ, Suico JG, et al. Units of measure in clinical information systems. J Am Med Inform Assoc 1999;6(2):151–62.

16. Flatman R. Terminology, units and reporting: how harmonized do we need to be? Clin Chem Lab Med 2018;57(1):1–11.

17. Gansel X, Mary M, van Belkum A. Semantic data interoperability, digital medicine, and e-health in infectious disease management: a review. Eur J Clin Microbiol Infect Dis 2019;38(6):1023–34.

18. Burger G, Abu-Hanna A, de Keizer N, et al. Natural language processing in pathology: a scoping review. J Clin Pathol 2016. https://doi.org/10.1136/jclinpath-2016-203872.

19. Bietenbeck A, Streichert T. Preparing laboratories for interconnected health care. Diagnostics (Basel) 2021;11(8):1487–94.

20. Van Cott EM. Laboratory test interpretations and algorithms in utilization management. Clin Chim Acta 2014;427:188–92.

21. Laposata ME, Laposata M, Van Cott EM, et al. Physician survey of a laboratory medicine interpretive service and evaluation of the influence of interpretations on laboratory test ordering. Arch Pathol Lab Med 2004;128(12):1424–7.

22. Vasikaran S, Sikaris K, Kilpatrick E, et al. Assuring the quality of interpretative comments in clinical chemistry. Clin Chem Lab Med 2016;54(12):1901–11.

23. Bezzegh A, Takács I, Ajzner É. Toward harmonization of interpretive commenting of common laboratory tests. Clin Biochem 2017;50(10–11):612–6.

24. Krumm N, Shirts BH. Technical, biological, and systems barriers for molecular clinical decision support. Clin Lab Med 2019;39(2):281–94.

25. Conway JR, et al. Next-generation sequencing and the clinical oncology workflow: data challenges, proposed solutions, and a call to action. JCO Precis Oncol 2019;3.

26. Nakhleh RE. Quality in surgical pathology communication and reporting. Arch Pathol Lab Med 2011;135(11):1394–7.

27. Srigley JR, McGowan T, Maclean A, et al. Standardized synoptic cancer pathology reporting: a population-based approach. J Surg Oncol 2009;99(8):517–24.

28. Campbell WS, Karlsson D, Vreeman DJ, et al. A computable pathology report for precision medicine: extending an observables ontology unifying SNOMED CT and LOINC. J Am Med Inform Assoc 2018;25(3):259–66.

29. Campbell WS, Campbell JR, West WW, et al. Semantic analysis of SNOMED CT for a post-coordinated database of histopathology findings. J Am Med Inform Assoc 2014;21(5):885–92.
30. Ayaz M, Pasha MF, Alzahrani MY, et al. The fast health interoperability resources (FHIR) standard: systematic literature review of implementations, applications, challenges and opportunities. JMIR Med Inform 2021;9(7):e21929.
31. Strasberg HR, Rhodes B, Del Fiol G, et al. Contemporary clinical decision support standards using health level seven international fast healthcare interoperability resources. J Am Med Inform Assoc 2021;28(8):1796–806.
32. Weber GM, Adams WG, Bernstam EV, et al. Biases introduced by filtering electronic health records for patients with "complete data". J Am Med Inform Assoc 2017;24(6):1134–41.
33. Luo Y, Szolovits P, Dighe AS, et al. 3D-MICE: integration of cross-sectional and longitudinal imputation for multi-analyte longitudinal clinical data. J Am Med Inform Assoc 2018;25(6):645–53.
34. Luo Y, Szolovits P, Dighe AS, et al. Using machine learning to predict laboratory test results. Am J Clin Pathol 2016;145(6):778–88.
35. Martin S, Wagner J, Lupulescu-Mann N, et al. Comparison of EHR-based diagnosis documentation locations to a gold standard for risk stratification in patients with multiple chronic conditions. Appl Clin Inform 2017;8(3):794–809.
36. Burrows EK, Razzaghi H, Utidjian L, et al. Standardizing clinical diagnoses: evaluating alternate terminology selection. AMIA Jt Summits Transl Sci Proc 2020; 2020:71–9.
37. Amos L, Anderson D, Brody S, et al. UMLS users and uses: a current overview. J Am Med Inform Assoc 2020;27(10):1606–11.
38. Wright A, McCoy AB, Hickman TT, et al. Problem list completeness in electronic health records: a multi-site study and assessment of success factors. Int J Med Inform 2015;84(10):784–90.
39. Reimer AP, Dai W, Smith B, et al. Subcategorizing EHR diagnosis codes to improve clinical application of machine learning models. Int J Med Inform 2021;156:104588.
40. Wright A, McGlinchey EA, Poon EG, et al. Ability to generate patient registries among practices with and without electronic health records. J Med Internet Res 2009;11(3):e31.
41. Schmittdiel J, Bodenheimer T, Solomon NA, et al. Brief report: the prevalence and use of chronic disease registries in physician organizations. A national survey. J Gen Intern Med 2005;20(9):855–8.
42. Johnson KE, Kamineni A, Fuller S, et al. How the provenance of electronic health record data matters for research: a case example using system mapping. EGEMS (Wash DC) 2014;2(1):1058.
43. Kelly J, Wang C, Zhang J, et al. Automated mapping of real-world oncology laboratory data to LOINC. AMIA Annu Symp Proc 2021;2021:611–20.

Clinical Artificial Intelligence
Design Principles and Fallacies

Matthew B.A. McDermott, PhD[a],*, Bret Nestor, MS[b],
Peter Szolovits, PhD[a]

KEYWORDS

- Artificial intelligence • Machine learning • Misspecification • Irresponsibility
- Uninterpretability

KEY POINTS

- Without careful consideration of the machine learning (ML)/artificial intelligence (AI) design process and the problem of interest, effective use of ML/AI in the clinic is challenged by several key problems.
- Model misspecification is when the evaluation process for an ML tool does not sufficiently mirror the real world, which can lead to significant problems when tools are deployed.
- Even when correctly specified, models must be developed responsibly, taking into consideration performance across numerous patient subpopulations and evaluation settings to ensure models are fair and unbiased.
- Tools from interpretability can help catch some of these issues before model deployment, but also pose challenges of their own and need to be used carefully.

INTRODUCTION

Clinical artificial intelligence (AI)/machine learning (ML) is anticipated to offer new abilities in clinical decision support, diagnostic reasoning, precision medicine, clinical operational support, and clinical research.[1–6] However, in practice, it is hard to determine how one can effectively use ML/AI techniques for real-world problems.[2,6] This confusion stems from various factors, including that: (1) ML for health is often explored in solely academic settings, without considering the nuances of true clinical deployments; (2) clinicians deploying ML algorithms in practice may have different backgrounds and have different stages of familiarity with ML methodology and assumptions than those in the research community; and (3) many nontechnical

[a] CSAIL, MIT, 32 Vassar St, Cambridge, MA 02139, USA; [b] Department of Computer Science, University of Toronto, 40 St George St, Toronto, ON M5S 2E4, Canada
* Corresponding author.
E-mail address: matthew_mcdermott@hms.harvard.edu

Clin Lab Med 43 (2023) 29–46
https://doi.org/10.1016/j.cll.2022.09.004
0272-2712/23/© 2022 Elsevier Inc. All rights reserved.
labmed.theclinics.com

barriers exist preventing the widespread use of ML in health care, limiting practical examples of its usage.

Ultimately, regardless of its cause, this uncertainty results in many real-world problems, such as the development and use of ML algorithms in inappropriate contexts, ML models demonstrating unexpectedly poor performance in deployment scenarios, and substantial disparities in algorithm performance across patient subpopulations.[2,7,8]

In this work, we provide a practical overview of clinical ML/AI designed to ameliorate some of these issues. We focus not on providing a technical overview into clinical ML, because such tutorials and resources are widely available elsewhere,[9–15] but rather on outlining the distinct aspects of clinical AI that give rise to common fallacies, which can hinder progress in this domain. By understanding these fallacies, clinician scientists will be able to develop stronger intuition regarding effective use of ML tools in health research and deployment and will be able to anticipate key issues in the deployment of ML/AI tools.

To elicit understanding of clinical ML/AI, we first delve into the design specifications of clinical ML/AI. We focus specifically on core questions that one must answer before beginning any ML project, and examples of ML applications within health care across medical imaging modalities, tabular electronic health record (EHR) data, and clinical text.

Next, we overview three key areas of common ML fallacies: (1) misspecification, that is, when models are inapplicable; (2) irresponsibility, that is, when models are misleading; and (3) uninterpretability, that is, when models are inexplicable. Within each area, we detail several concrete kinds of problems clinicians are likely to encounter, and how to approach addressing these problems. Finally, we close with concluding thoughts.

CLINICAL MACHINE LEARNING AND ARTIFICIAL INTELLIGENCE
What Is Machine Learning/Artificial Intelligence?

ML is the process of designing a computational algorithm to reason about data. This process can take many forms, including classical examples, such as linear or logistic regression models, survival models, tree-based models, Gaussian processes, and nearest neighbor models, and more recently prominent examples, such as deep neural network models, including feed-forward, convolutional, recurrent, or transformer neural networks. For further technical details on the kinds of ML models one can use, interested readers should refer to existing review articles or other online tutorials.[9–15] Note that for the purposes of this work, we take the terms "machine learning" and "artificial intelligence" to be synonyms, and by convention we generally use the term "machine learning."

Machine Learning Problem Setup

General framing
In considering whether an ML tool can be used to help solve a problem in a clinical context, it is important to first understand how to frame problems as "ML problems" in general.

Typically, an ML problem begins with a dataset X (eg, a collection of medical images, patient laboratory test results, free-text notes, or any combination of these modalities). We often assume the data X is drawn as a collection of independent, random samples x_i from some probability distribution p_X: $x_i \sim p$.

For supervised ML problems, we also have some target Y that we want to classify (eg, the patient's likelihood of having a certain diagnosis). Then, the ML task is to design a model, denoted as f, realized as a mathematical function which is often parameterized by some numerical parameters θ drawn from some space of possible parameters Θ, which is capable of mapping the input data-points x_i to their appropriate output label with high fidelity: $f_\theta^*: x_i \rightarrow \tilde{y}_i$, with $\tilde{y}_i$ approximating y_i. The function f (or more typically, the optimal parameters θ^* for f) is often learned through an iterative training process, where the parameters are locally optimized in each iteration to improve some objective function measured on the training data. This objective function is chosen to quantify the difference between the prediction $\tilde{y}_i$ and the true label y_i, and to regularize some measure of the complexity of the model (eg, the number of nonzero parameters in θ^*) to ensure strong generalizability.

To put this framing in context, consider learning a statistical version of an early warning score, such as the NEWS score for sepsis.[16] The "model" f takes as input features a patient's respiratory rate, oxygen saturation, and all other categories leveraged by the NEWS scores. Its parameters θ are integers corresponding to the penalties given for each variable category in the score (eg, the model would have a parameter corresponding to the additive effect of a respiratory rate ≤ 8, which in the published model is +3). Finally, we would judge its efficacy via an objective function quantifying the extent to which a higher risk score in a patient is associated with increased risk of sepsis via retrospective data.

At deployment time, only the final, optimized model f_θ^* is used, and naturally true labels are generally not known. Furthermore, real-world impact of the ML system will typically be judged via a different procedure than that used to evaluate the model during training, such as the extent to which patient outcomes improve after integrating the risk score into the clinical workflow.

Key design questions
Among the many questions that arise during the development of a clinical ML tool, here we highlight three key questions that can help ensure success in the clinic of the resulting ML/AI tool.

1. What problem are you solving (and how do you determine success)?
   a. What problem, conceptually, are you trying to solve, and how would a model capable of reasoning over data help solve it?
   b. What does it mean for $\tilde{y}_i$ to approximate y? How can you tell if a model is good enough for use in the desired application?
   c. How reflective is your development output label Y of the true deployment task you intend to solve?
2. What does your data look like?
   a. What is the modality of the input X (eg, images, tabular data, narrative text, waveforms)? Is/should the input data be static or temporal in nature?
   b. What is the modality of the output Y (eg, categorical, numerical)?
   c. How much training data do you have available, and how much of that training data is labeled? How much coverage of your input domain do you have within your dataset (eg, are there patient subpopulations or labels that are underrepresented)?
3. What kind of model do you want to learn?
   a. What are the expectations you would have around the resulting function f? Would you expect a linear function to perform well? Or are the relationships here expected to be nonlinear in nature?
   b. What constraints do you want to place on the model f_θ^*? Should it conform to certain clinical expectations?

   c. What trade-offs are acceptable in final performance to ensure your model and parameters obey the desired constraints?

Appropriate consideration to these questions greatly speeds up the process of ML model development and increases the likelihood that the eventual model is useful for the targeted deployment. A visual overview of this entire design process, along with where these key questions fit into that framework, is found in **Fig. 1**.

Other kinds of machine learning problem setups
In the framing provided previously, an ML problem is presented as being defined via an input dataset X and target labels Y. However, in reality, this framing only naively applies to traditional classification or regression problems. There also exist numerous other kinds of ML problems, such as clustering, where the only input is the dataset X, and the learning task is to identify appropriate groupings (eg, clusters) of datapoints in X; reinforcement learning, where the dataset X contains histories of decisions made and (via some metric) outcomes of those decisions, such that the model is trained to learn an optimal decision-making policy; or imputation, where the input is a dataset X with some measurements unknown, and the objective is to learn a model that can impute these missing entries most accurately.

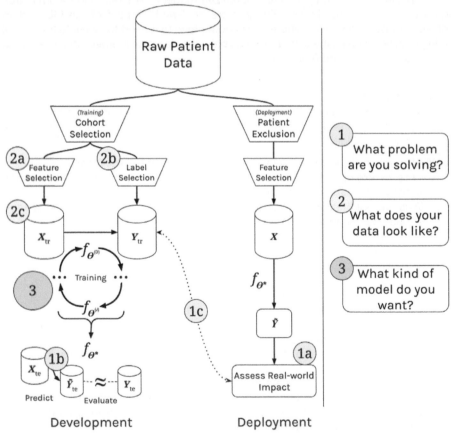

Fig. 1. A visual overview of the ML design process, highlighting where the three key questions come up in this representation.

Important Machine Learning Terms for Clinicians

Generalizability

In designing an ML model, one must carefully consider how to leverage the available data to produce the best result not during the training/evaluation process itself, but rather during the eventual deployment of the ultimate model to the real-world setting. This is ultimately a question of generalizability, which refers to the extent to which a model's performance on a training dataset X_{tr} can be expected to reflect the performance in various deployment scenarios.

Generalizability, in reality, encompasses two concerns: whether or not the evaluation of the final model f_{θ}^* is statistically identical to evaluating f_{θ}^* on a new, randomly sampled dataset $X_{tr} \sim p$; and whether or not this evaluation result is statistically identical to the evaluation that would be obtained in the final deployment environment. These two concerns are important, but are also different. The first typically is fully addressed through appropriate statistical methodology during model development. The second concern, however, is much more challenging to address, because in many cases model developers do not have sufficient information to appropriately model the true deployment setting. Selection criteria in crafting the training cohort X, Y may not be mirrored in the general population, for example, and important patient subpopulations may not have labels measured at all.

Capacity

The capacity of an ML model class is colloquially used to reflect the complexity of the kinds of functions that model class can learn to reflect. For example, linear models (eg, linear regression, logistic regression, linear support vector machines/support vector classifiers, Cox proportional hazard) can only reflect linear relationships between their inputs (eg, covariates, independent variables) and their outputs (eg, response variables, dependent variables, or the log-likelihood of said), and are therefore low capacity.

In contrast, such methods as ensemble methods (eg, random forests, extremely boosted trees), neural networks, nearest neighbor methods, and others are high-capacity methods capable of modeling much richer function classes. Deep neural networks, in particular, are known to be capable of approximating any arbitrary function to high-fidelity, provided they are sufficiently deep and wide. Of course, commensurate with their increased capabilities, higher-capacity models also have several major drawbacks, including much higher requirements on training data, computational resources, and energy expenditure; increased risk of overfitting or sensitivity to dataset noise; and substantially reduced interpretability versus lower capacity methods. Accordingly, it is imperative to always assess the efficacy of simpler, low-capacity techniques in modeling contexts even when high-capacity models may ultimately offer better performance.

Causality

Much like traditional statistical analysis, ML models can either be causal or strictly correlative in nature. And, also much like traditional statistics, in general ML models will be correlative and should not be assumed to offer any causal insight. Causal inference is an active field of study across traditional statistics and ML, and there are several techniques that permit drawing causal insights, even only over retrospective data, including casual models and reinforcement learning.

In health contexts, where we may imagine integrating ML systems into clinical workflows, it is paramount to understand if the techniques used are appropriate to the kind of inference you intend to draw from the associated model. Even beyond typical concerns of correlation versus causation, in clinical decision support contexts, ML models may taint their own future training data with their current recommendations, so these concerns must be carefully examined in any continuous deployment setting.

Examples of Machine Learning Problems in Health

ML techniques have been used in various areas within health and biomedicine. In this section, we highlight several specific areas, but interested readers should consult various other reviews for a more detailed description of the variety of research conducted in this field.[2,17–19]

Machine learning for medical imaging

One prevalent area for ML in health care is in the analysis of medical images (eg, radiographs, pathology slides).[19–21] Here, we highlight several specific research areas within ML for medical imaging, spanning deployed and nondeployed settings.

Diagnostic classification of chest radiographs. One major area of ML for health research is in the automatic diagnosis and modeling of chest radiographs. Motivated by major benchmarks including CheXpert,[22] MIMIC-CXR,[23] and the NIH Chest X-ray 14 dataset,[24] numerous works have explored using convolutional neural networks to automatically diagnose patients via chest radiographs alone.[25,26]

However, these works also suffer from several major concerns that have inhibited deployment of tools based on these models. In particular, it is well documented that classifiers in this space have major fairness and bias concerns.[27–29] Furthermore, the diagnostic labels used for training for many of these models itself are often automatically determined via natural language processing (NLP) tools and suffer from notable inaccuracies.[22,23] Overall, additional research is needed to determine if these efforts will translate into substantial improvements for real patients in the clinic.

Diagnostic classification of diabetic retinopathy. Another prominent area within ML for medical imaging is in the detection of diabetic retinopathy via fundus images. This work is particularly motivated by the major shortage of qualified providers and the significant burden of diabetic retinopathy globally. However, even in this area, which attracts extensive corporate investment and has produced models that work extremely well during development, deployment efforts have found major sociotechnical challenges limiting patient impact.[30,31]

Successfully deployed imaging-based machine learning tools. Despite some of the challenges mentioned in prior paragraphs, there are a large number of ML tools approved for use in practice in medical imaging today (eg, https://grand-challenge.org/aiforradiology/). However, despite the large number of approved projects, as of 2021 only approximately 18% of approved products had prospectively demonstrated clinical impact.[32] This does not only reflect the difficulty in bridging the laboratory-clinic divide, but it is also worth noting that many deployed software avoid addressing diagnostic/therapeutic tasks in lieu of operational tasks, such as image segmentation, quantification, or structured data extraction.[32]

Machine learning for structured, numerical electronic health record data

Another common target for ML in health care is the analysis of structured EHR data, such as patients' laboratory test results, vital signs, and physician ordering behaviors. Here, we highlight several key areas for research and deployment leveraging tabular EHR data.

Research into various clinical benchmark tasks for machine learning model development. Because of the availability of large, public, EHR datasets for ML,[23,33] there are myriad research articles targeting various clinical tasks without clear deployment targets. These include, for example, mortality prediction, ICD code classification, intervention response prediction, and imputation of laboratory values, among others.[34–38] It is also well established that these models suffer from concerns regarding generalizability/robustness,[39] fairness/bias,[40,41] and applicability to true clinical tasks.[2,3] Nonetheless, despite these concerns and that these models have rarely been integrated into deployed clinical solutions, these tasks have enabled research into ML techniques for EHR data.

Deployed systems. One notable example of a clinical ML product deployed for patient care management is Duke University's Sepsis Watch program. This program consists of a fully deployed, real-world assessment of a sepsis prediction and management system based on ML models.[42–44]

Ultimately, researchers on this study have noted that the deployment process necessitated extensive work above and beyond the technical and model development work, including stakeholder alignment and trust-building, careful integration into real clinical workflows, and careful evaluation of the tool to assess bias across subpopulations. This work also resulted in a clinical trial designed to assess the impact on actual patient care of the Sepsis Watch program. Although this clinical trial concluded in July of 2019, as of now (May 2022) there have been no follow-up studies detailing the findings of this clinical trial.[45]

Another example of ML systems leveraging structured EHR data being successfully deployed is the Oravizio system for predicting risks for joint replacement surgery. The developers of this system have noted the importance of certain software development principles, the availability of data, and continuous training systems in the process of the deployment of their system.[46]

Hospital operational support via patient flow management. There are also several ML systems in use in hospitals today to help manage the operational aspects of health care. Of particular note are patient flow management solutions, which leverage data science and ML tools to better forecast patient flow, including length-of-stay, discharge, and readmission risk prediction. In these areas, there has been ample research investment[47,48] and there are several deployed solutions that are already in use.[49,50]

Machine learning for clinical text

The final area we highlight in this review is the use of NLP for the analysis of clinical narrative text.[51–53] Here, we find that despite ample research investment, there are proportionally even fewer instances of deployed tools leveraging these techniques. We focus primarily on two areas: the use of NLP for structured data extraction from narrative text; and the use of NLP for text-generation applications, such as question answering, summarization, or dialogue generation.

Structured data extraction via natural language processing. In the clinical NLP research field, one common suite of tasks entails structured data extraction from narrative text. This includes such tasks as named entity recognition (eg, identification of symptoms or diseases),[54–56] relation extraction (eg, identifying assertions of disease-symptom or disease-treatment relationships),[57–59] or temporal context identification (eg, identifying the temporal ordering of presented symptoms in narrative notes).[60]

These systems have been used in offline, information retrieval applications, and to facilitate further research themselves, but have limited direct clinical deployment themselves.

Text generation applications: Question answering, summarization, translation, and dialogue. More complex clinical NLP tasks often involve some aspect of text generation. Although this area has advanced tremendously in the general domain (eg, the raw generative capabilities of the GPT series language models[61] or the question-answering abilities of the T0pp model[62] are quite impressive) similar advancements in the clinical domain have yet to be fully realized. This is not to say numerous examples of these kinds of tasks do not exist in clinical NLP; indeed, research has explored tasks ranging from radiology report generation,[63,64] automatic summarization of medical records,[65,66] medical question-answering,[67,68] and medical translation tasks.[69] Despite these studies, however, clinical NLP has yet to demonstrate successes at the level of those seen in the general domain, and these methods are not typically yet deployed in patient facing applications.

One notable area where text-generation solutions are being deployed for patient use is in the development of various medical chat-bot applications. Although such methods have a storied history (eg, the ELIZA model[70]) in more recent times, various companies have begun exploring these technologies for consumer-facing medical applications.[71] Given the novelty of these technologies, more time is needed to see if these companies ultimately provide value to patients.

CLINICAL ARTIFICIAL INTELLIGENCE FALLACIES

In the previous section, we explored the ML design process and overviewed a diverse set of clinical ML methods in academia and in deployment. Throughout that exploration, we highlighted various common points of concern and barriers to effective deployment for ML methods in the clinic. In this section, we crystallize these concerns, and in particular discuss three concrete, common mistakes in the development and deployment of ML models for health applications, and strategies to address them, or even to avoid them altogether.

In particular, we first discuss various forms of model misspecification, when the design of a model differs sufficiently from its eventual deployment setting that poor deployment performance is likely. Next, we discuss risks of irresponsibility in clinical ML; when models, even models trained correctly, can result in harm to patients at deployment time because of preventable factors. Finally, we close this section discussing interpretability, and when and how interpretability-driven analyses can aid or hinder model development and deployment in health settings.

Misspecification: When Models Are Inapplicable

Misspecification relates principally to question one in the list of key design questions defined previously: What is your problem and how do you measure success? In particular, here we use the term "misspecification" to reflect any discrepancies between how models are trained and evaluated during the development process versus how they will actually be used at deployment time. Next, we discuss three different kinds of misspecification in more detail.

Performance measures on paper versus in the clinic
The first form of misspecification we cover is a simple, but surprisingly common issue in clinical ML: when the evaluation process used during model design does not appropriately reflect the concerns relevant to the ultimate deployment use-case.[6] For example, many models in the academic literature are evaluated using metrics well suited for model comparison, such as the area under the receiver operating characteristic.[35,39] However, in practice, we rarely care about such metrics directly, at least as

compared with more specialized, targeted metrics, such as quantifications of patient harm, underdiagnosis or misdiagnosis rate, or reduction in health care cost.

Of course, there are many works that do use more targeted evaluation metrics for their ultimate use cases, including partial area under the receiver operating characteristic,[72] direct underdiagnosis rates,[27] and many others. However, it is nonetheless challenging to design evaluation metrics that are at once suitable for training and fully reflective of the ultimate deployment use case.

Therefore, when considering ML solutions for health problems, researchers should think carefully about how their model will ultimately be used in practice, what metrics are critical in that setting, and how those can be best approximated during development. An excellent example of this fallacy in action is in the rampant proliferation of ML-based COVID screening and triage tools. Although many such tools have demonstrated excellent performance during development, critics argue that none have actually yielded clinically meaningful improvements to care practices, and that many are not even safe to deploy today.[73,74]

Generalizability gaps
Beyond direct technical misspecification, models often also face issues relating to generalizability when transitioning from a development to a deployment setting. For example, if a model is developed based on the population from hospital A, but is ultimately deployed for use at hospital B, the differences in the underlying patient populations, care practices, data encoding systems, and more between A and B can result in significant degradation in performance.[75]

Ultimately, some amount of domain shift is, in practice, unavoidable.[76] If nothing else, models will always be trained on historical data, but deployed on future data, which itself represents some form of population shift.[77] Although it may seem minor, this temporal drift can pose a serious problem,[39] especially because hospital care practices/data encoding strategies change over time. This problem is compounded if a model is actually deployed in such a manner that it then affects future data directly (eg, by influencing physician behavior). In this setting, continual training regimes, a common solution to account for temporal drift, will now be much noisier because of the model's influence on its own future training data, and specialized algorithms that can address these temporal dynamics (eg, reinforcement learning) should be considered.[78]

In general, model developers should carefully interrogate (1) how extensive these domain shifts are likely to be, (2) if training/development procedures can be modified to assess this generalizability gap,[79–81] and (3) if the model class (eg, high-capacity or low-capacity) is likely to be robust to population shifts in deployment settings.

Confounders
A particular form of generalizability gaps that warrant specific attention are those motivated by unknown or unobserved confounders. In particular, it is common, especially in correlative modeling settings, that model performance during development may be driven primarily by factors that do not causally relate to the expected clinical pathways of interest in deployment. For example, models can rely on signals indicating a patient is being treated for a specific disease to identify the diagnosis of that disease,[82] or it may rely on clinician behavior to motivate an erroneously low-risk score.[83,84] In such settings, models can show high performance at training time, but then induce harm when deployed in real-world settings because the signals they learned to rely on at training time no longer apply in the real-world setting.

Interpretability tools can help model developers interrogate the factors of their data that help drive model performance in the training setting, which can ultimately reveal these problematic noncausal associations.

Irresponsibility: When Models Are Misleading

Even when models are correctly specified, insufficient or irresponsible interrogation of model design and evaluation can mask profound risks of patient harm during deployment. These concerns reflect aspects spanning all three key design questions. In this section, we highlight two key areas exemplifying these risks.

Fairness and bias

The first concern we need to highlight here is the risk that clinical ML models can provide disparate performance across patient subgroups and/or exacerbate existing health inequalities. There are numerous examples of this in today's literature, including studies showing that diagnostic classifiers trained on chest radiograph exhibit significant disparities across race, gender, and insurance type subgroups[27,28]; that clinical language models automatically encode racial biases simply via underlying training text[85]; and that already deployed models exhibit significant racial disparities because of misattribution of health care costs as health needs,[7] among others.[40,86]

Note that these examples all stem from numerous factors affecting different portions of the design process. For example, one's dataset can be biased or misattributed,[7] one's training procedure can exacerbate existing biases in the underlying clinical data,[27,87] and one's evaluation procedure can mask concerns about disparities via population statistics.[85]

Appropriately accounting for concerns of the risk of bias in clinical ML is challenging. At the very least, model developers should assess performance across diverse and intersectional patient subpopulations and speak with domain experts to ensure the underlying model assumptions are not themselves inherently biased (eg, that outcome proxies are not likely to be less appropriate for patient subgroups).[88] Interested readers can consult a review of this area[41] for further insights into ensuring that trained models take appropriate steps to address this issue.

Reproducibility

Even when accounting for all other issues, model results may simply not be reproducible. This is true even when all best practices are followed, and in general it is well documented that ML4H suffers from ample issues w.r.t. reproducibility.[89] Unfortunately, presuming the other steps outlined in this work are taken, there are no easy solutions to ensure a model is likely to fully reproduce to a deployment environment. As a result, model deployment should always be performed in a responsible, careful manner that involves thorough human evaluation, and regular model audits to ensure performance remains stable even over time as the underlying data distributions shift.[90]

Uninterpretability: When Models Are Inexplicable

As soon as a clinical ML model reaches suitable performance, stakeholders wonder how to appropriately interpret the results. Interpretability is often stated as being a requirement to build trust among stakeholders in model performance, and it is further often asserted that specific techniques can be used to gain interpretability, such as the use of saliency maps, feature sensitivity analyses, or maximal activation signals.[91–94] However, these views are also contested, with critics arguing that interpretability is an ill-defined notion, with definitions often in conflict with one another, and that the requirement of a model being interpretable to build trust among stakeholders is artificial.[95,96]

Although these critiques are valid, interpretability techniques have been used in practice as an invaluable tool for validating that a model is leveraging appropriate causal pathways to drive its decisions. For example, while developing a model predicting mortality risk for patients with tuberculosis, Caruana and colleagues[83] leveraged an interpretable model type (in particular through human evaluation of learned rule-sets) to discover that their model was (incorrectly) predicting that patients suffering from asthma and tuberculosis were at lower risk for severe disease. This phenomenon was ultimately discovered to be caused by a causal misalignment of the prediction task and desired use case,[83] because the model was not taking into account that patients with asthma and tuberculosis were naturally treated more aggressively by clinicians from the outset, and thus were only demonstrating superior outcomes because of this increased treatment. Similarly, Oakden-Rayner and colleagues[82] have leveraged interpretability techniques (in particular error auditing) to detect the hidden clinical stratification in models trained to predict a patient's diagnosis via chest radiographs.

Despite these successes, model developers must be careful when leveraging interpretability techniques as a validation tool, especially for high-capacity models.[97] This is because, much like any form of statistical analysis, without careful consideration, it is easy to misattribute interpretability signals to underlying model properties solely based on spurious signals. In reality, model performance often is inexplicable (eg, recent results have demonstrated that models are capable of predicting a patient's race from a chest radiograph, despite that model developers and clinical experts alike cannot determine how the model is able to form this prediction[29]) and if one's method of examining interpretability signals does not permit that as a possible result, it is inherently a biased form of model validation. In addition, studies have shown that model interpretability can also inhibit a user's ability to recognize when the model makes errors, which is often counter to the purpose of including interpretability studies.[98]

To help combat this bias and ensure interpretability techniques help improve model validation, users should consider the following questions when deploying these tools:

1. Can you codify your expectations regarding what should drive model performance (and, importantly, what should not drive performance) before beginning interpretability analysis? Much like preregistering the outcome of a clinical trial, identifying one's hypotheses before investigating model interpretations can help limit spurious findings.

2. Have you considered the impact multilinearity (eg, feature-feature correlation) and more general feature interdependence can have on interpretability results? For example, interpretability weightings may be split or masked across many interrelated features, and conversely false signals can also appear more heavily weighted if anticorrelated features are also leveraged heavily.

3. Is it possible the model can predict unexpected patient covariates from the presented information that could further inform final outcomes? If so, then even if these covariates are excluded, they may still be having a significant impact on model results in undesired ways.

4. Are the interpretability methods used capable of detecting the kinds of relationships you anticipate? For example, simply examining feature importance weights independently cannot be used to inform you if the model is leveraging groups of features in nonlinear manners. Similarly, examining population-level error statistics (or static model features) cannot help determine what drives a model's prediction for an individual sample in the dataset.

SUMMARY

In this work, we (1) outline the design process of clinical ML/AI tools; (2) identify several key design questions one must consider when developing such a tool, including understanding what is your problem, what does your data look like, and what kind of model do you want; and (3) highlight several common sources of issues in deployed clinical ML/AI technologies, including misspecification, irresponsibility, and uninterpretability. Alongside each of these, we also present concrete examples of ML/AI tools in health care, at the research/development stage and (where possible) deployed in clinical practice.

Through this careful consideration of the design landscape here, it is hoped that this work can help the ML for health community develop stronger intuition regarding effective use and deployment of ML tools and better enable these practices to ultimately help patients and physicians.

CLINICS CARE POINTS

- ML Models must be carefully evaluated prior to use in the clinic.
- Users of ML tools must carefully consider whether their use case is aligned with the manner in which the tool was evaluated, and whether or not the population of interest is well represented in the model's evaluation set.
- When using interpretability tools to assess model validity, users must be careful to perform an unbiased assessment of the model.

DISCLOSURE

This work is funded in part by National Institutes of Health, United States grant LM013337 and by a collaborative research agreement with IBM. The authors have no additional financial agreements to disclose.

REFERENCES

1. Yu KH, Beam AL, Kohane IS. Artificial intelligence in healthcare. Nat Biomed Eng 2018;2(10):719–31.
2. Ghassemi M, Naumann T, Schulam P, et al. A review of challenges and opportunities in machine learning for health. AMIA Summits Transl Sci Proc 2020; 2020:191.
3. Kelly CJ, Karthikesalingam A, Suleyman M, et al. Key challenges for delivering clinical impact with artificial intelligence. BMC Med 2019;17:195.
4. Davenport T, Kalakota R. The potential for artificial intelligence in healthcare. Future Healthc J 2019;6(2):94–8.
5. Miotto R, Wang F, Wang S, et al. Deep learning for healthcare: review, opportunities and challenges. Brief Bioinform 2018;19(6):1236–46.
6. Wiens J, Saria S, Sendak M, et al. Do no harm: a roadmap for responsible machine learning for health care. Nat Med 2019;25(9):1337–40.
7. Obermeyer Z, Powers B, Vogeli C, et al. Dissecting racial bias in an algorithm used to manage the health of populations. Science 2019;366(6464):447–53.
8. Ghassemi M, Mohamed S. Machine learning and health need better values. NPJ Digital Med 2022;5(1):1–4.

9. Arbet J, Brokamp C, Meinzen-Derr J, et al. Lessons and tips for designing a machine learning study using EHR data. J Clin Translational Sci 2021;5(1).

10. Shen L, Kann BH, Taylor RA, et al. The clinician's guide to the machine learning galaxy. Front Physiol 2021;12:658583.

11. Esteva A, Robicquet A, Ramsundar B, et al. A guide to deep learning in healthcare. Nat Med 2019;25(1):24–9.

12. Rowe M. An introduction to machine learning for clinicians. Acad Med 2019; 94(10):1433–6.

13. Fundamentals of machine learning for healthcare. Coursera. Available at: https://www.coursera.org/learn/fundamental-machine-learning-healthcare. Accessed June 10, 2022.

14. AI in healthcare. Coursera. Available at: https://www.coursera.org/specializations/ai-healthcare. Accessed June 10, 2022.

15. Ahmad MA, Eckert C, Teredesai A. Interpretable machine learning in healthcare. In: Proceedings of the 2018 ACM International Conference on Bioinformatics, Computational Biology, and Health Informatics. BCB '18. Association for Computing Machinery; 2018:559–560.

16. Smith GB, Redfern OC, Pimentel MAF, et al. The national early warning score 2 (NEWS2). Clinical medicine. J R Coll Physicians Lond 2019;19(3):260.

17. Nayyar A, Gadhavi L, Zaman N. Machine learning in healthcare: review, opportunities and challenges. Machine Learn Internet Med Things Healthc 2021;23–45.

18. Shailaja K, Seetharamulu B, Jabbar MA. Machine learning in healthcare: a review. In: 2018 Second International Conference on Electronics, Communication and Aerospace Technology (ICECA). IEEE; 2018:910–914.

19. Varoquaux G, Cheplygina V. Machine learning for medical imaging: methodological failures and recommendations for the future. NPJ digital Med 2022;5(1):1–8.

20. Zhou SK, Greenspan H, Davatzikos C, et al. A review of deep learning in medical imaging: imaging traits, technology trends, case studies with progress highlights, and future promises. Proc IEEE 2021;109:820–38.

21. Aggarwal R, Sounderajah V, Martin G, et al. Diagnostic accuracy of deep learning in medical imaging: a systematic review and meta-analysis. NPJ digital Med 2021;4(1):1–23.

22. Irvin J., Rajpurkar P., Ko M., et al. Chexpert: A large chest radiograph dataset with uncertainty labels and expert comparison. In: Proceedings of the AAAI Conference on Artificial Intelligence, Honolulu, HI. Vol 33, 1/27/2019 - 2/1/2019, 590–597.

23. Johnson AEW, Pollard TJ, Shen L, et al. MIMIC-III, a freely accessible critical care database. Scientific data 2016;3(1):1–9.

24. Wang X., Peng Y., Lu L., et al. Chestx-ray8: Hospital-scale chest x-ray database and benchmarks on weakly-supervised classification and localization of common thorax diseases. In: Proceedings of the IEEE Conference on Computer Vision and Pattern Recognition, Honolulu, HI. 7/22/2017 - 7/25/2017, 2097–2106.

25. Rajpurkar P, Irvin J, Zhu K, et al. Chexnet: radiologist-level pneumonia detection on chest x-rays with deep learning. arXiv 2017. https://doi.org/10.48550/arXiv.1711.05225.

26. Allaouzi I, Ahmed MB. A novel approach for multi-label chest X-ray classification of common thorax diseases. IEEE Access 2019;7:64279–88.

27. Seyyed-Kalantari L, Zhang H, McDermott M, et al. Underdiagnosis bias of artificial intelligence algorithms applied to chest radiographs in under-served patient populations. Nat Med 2021;27(12):2176–82.

28. Seyyed-Kalantari L., Liu G., McDermott M., et al. CheXclusion: fairness gaps in deep chest X-ray classifiers. In: BIOCOMPUTING 2021: Proceedings of the pacific Symposium. World Scientific; 2020:232–243. Availabe at: https://www.atsjournals.org/doi/epdf/10.1164/ajrccm-conference.2018.197.1_MeetingAbstracts.A3299.

29. Gichoya JW, Banerjee I, Bhimireddy AR, et al. AI recognition of patient race in medical imaging: a modelling study. The Lancet Digital Health 2022;4(6): E406–14.

30. Tsiknakis N, Theodoropoulos D, Manikis G, et al. Deep learning for diabetic retinopathy detection and classification based on fundus images: a review. Comput Biol Med 2021;135:104599.

31. Beede E, Baylor E, Hersch F, et al. A human-centered evaluation of a deep learning system deployed in clinics for the detection of diabetic retinopathy. In: Proceedings of the 2020 CHI Conference on Human Factors in Computing Systems. ; 2020:1–12.

32. van Leeuwen KG, Schalekamp S, Rutten MJ, et al. Artificial intelligence in radiology: 100 commercially available products and their scientific evidence. Eur Radiol 2021;31(6):3797–804.

33. Pollard TJ, Johnson AEW, Raffa JD, et al. The eICU Collaborative Research Database, a freely available multi-center database for critical care research. Scientific Data 2018;5(1):1–13.

34. McDermott M., Yan T., Naumann T., et al. Semi-supervised biomedical translation with cycle wasserstein regression GANs. In: Proceedings of the AAAI Conference on Artificial Intelligence, New Orleans, LA. Vol 32. 2/2/2018 - 2/7/2018.

35. McDermott M., Nestor B., Kim E., et al. A comprehensive EHR timeseries pretraining benchmark. In: Proceedings of the Conference on Health, Inference, and Learning (Virtual). 4/8/2021 - 4/10/2021, 257–278.

36. Suresh H, Hunt N, Johnson A, Celi LA, Szolovits P, Ghassemi M. Clinical intervention prediction and understanding with deep neural networks. In: Machine Learning for Healthcare Conference. PMLR; 2017:322–337.

37. Lipton ZC, Kale DC, Elkan C, et al. Learning to diagnose with LSTM recurrent neural networks. arXiv 2015. https://doi.org/10.48550/arXiv.1511.03677.

38. Yoon J, Jordon J, van der Schaar M. GAIN: Missing Data Imputation using generative adversarial nets. In: Dy JG, Krause A, eds Proceedings of the 35th International Conference on Machine Learning, ICML 2018, Stockholmsmässan, Stockholm, Sweden, July 10-15, 2018. Vol 80. Proceedings of Machine Learning Research. PMLR; 2018:5675-5684.

39. Nestor B, McDermott MBA, Boag W, et al. Feature robustness in non-stationary health records: caveats to deployable model performance in common clinical machine learning tasks. In: Doshi-Velez F, Fackler J, Jung K, et al., eds Proceedings of the 4th Machine Learning for Healthcare Conference. Vol 106. Proceedings of Machine Learning Research. PMLR; 09–10 Aug 2019:381–405.

40. Chen I, Johansson FD, Sontag D. Why is my classifier discriminatory?. In: Bengio S, Wallach H, Larochelle H, et al, editors. Advances in neural information processing systems, 31 Curran Associates, Inc; 2018. Available at: https://proceedings.neurips.cc/paper/2018/file/1f1baa5b8edac74eb4eaa329f14a0361-Paper.pdf.

41. Chen IY, Pierson E, Rose S, et al. Ethical machine learning in healthcare. Annu Rev Biomed Data Sci 2021;4(1):123–44.

42. Futoma J, Hariharan S, Heller K, et al. An improved multi-output gaussian process rnn with real-time validation for early sepsis detection. In: Machine Learning for Healthcare Conference. PMLR; 2017:243–254.

43. Futoma J, Hariharan S, Heller K. Learning to detect sepsis with a multitask Gaussian process RNN classifier. In: International Conference on Machine Learning. PMLR; 2017:1174–1182.

44. Lin AL, Sendak M, Bedoya A, et al. What is sepsis: investigating the heterogeneity of patient populations captured by different sepsis definitions. In: B43. Critical care: i still haven't found what i'm looking for-identifying and managing sepsis. American Thoracic Society; 2018. p. A3299.

45. Sendak MP, Ratliff W, Sarro D, et al. Real-world integration of a sepsis deep learning technology into routine clinical care: implementation study. JMIR Med Inform 2020;8(7):e15182.

46. Granlund T, Stirbu V, Mikkonen T. Towards regulatory-compliant mlops: oravizio's journey from a machine learning experiment to a deployed certified medical product. SN Computer Sci 2021;2(5):342.

47. El-Bouri R, Taylor T, Youssef A, et al. Machine learning in patient flow: a review. Prog Biomed Eng 2021;3(2):022002.

48. Stone K, Zwiggelaar R, Jones P, et al. A systematic review of the prediction of hospital length of stay: towards a unified framework. PLoS Digital Health 2022; 1(4):e0000017.

49. How we revolutionize the operational management of hospitals with Calyps AI. CALYPS. 2021. Available at: https://www.calyps.ch/en/how-we-revolutionize-the-operational-management-of-hospitals-with-calyps-ai/. Accessed May 16, 2022.

50. Healthcare Becker's. Qventus. How Boston Medical Center uses automation for early discharge planning. Becker's Health IT. 2022. https://www.beckershospitalreview.com/healthcare-information-technology/how-boston-medical-center-uses-automation-for-early-discharge-planning.html. Accessed May 16, 2022.

51. Wu S, Roberts K, Datta S, et al. Deep learning in clinical natural language processing: a methodical review. J Am Med Inform Assoc 2020;27(3):457–70.

52. Spasic I, Nenadic G. Others. Clinical text data in machine learning: systematic review. JMIR Med Inform 2020;8(3):e17984.

53. Le Glaz A, Haralambous Y, Kim-Dufor DH, et al. Machine learning and natural language processing in mental health: systematic review. J Med Internet Res 2021; 23(5):e15708.

54. Henry S, Wang Y, Shen F, et al. The 2019 National Natural language processing (NLP) Clinical Challenges (n2c2)/Open Health NLP (OHNLP) shared task on clinical concept normalization for clinical records. J Am Med Inform Assoc 2020; 27(10):1529–37. https://doi.org/10.1093/jamia/ocaa106.

55. Smit A, Jain S, Rajpurkar P, et al. Combining Automatic Labelers and Expert Annotations for Accurate Radiology Report Labeling Using BERT. Proceedings of the 2020 Conference on Empirical Methods in Natural Language Processing (EMNLP) 2020;117:1500–19.

56. McDermott MBA, Hsu TMH, Weng WH, Ghassemi M, Szolovits P. CheXpert++: approximating the CheXpert labeler for speed, differentiability, and probabilistic output. In: Doshi-Velez F, Fackler J, Jung K, et al., eds Proceedings of the 5th Machine Learning for Healthcare Conference. Vol 126. Proceedings of Machine Learning Research. PMLR; 07–08 Aug 2020:913–927.

57. Chauhan G, McDermott M, Szolovits P. Reflex: flexible framework for relation extraction in multiple domains. Proceedings of the 18th BioNLP Workshop and Shared Task 2019;W19-5004:30–47.

58. Roy A, Pan S. Incorporating medical knowledge in BERT for clinical relation extraction. In: Proceedings of the 2021 Conference on Empirical Methods in Natural Language Processing. ; 2021:5357–5366.

59. Wei Q, Ji Z, Si Y, et al. Relation extraction from clinical narratives using pre-trained language models. In: AMIA Annual Symposium Proceedings. Vol 2019. American Medical Informatics Association; 2019:1236.

60. Sun W, Rumshisky A, Uzuner O. Evaluating temporal relations in clinical text: 2012 i2b2 challenge. J Am Med Inform Assoc 2013;20(5):806–13.

61. Brown T, Mann B, Ryder N, et al. Language models are few-shot learners. Adv Neural Inf Process Syst 2020;33:1877–901.

62. Sanh V, Webson A, Raffel C, et al. Multitask prompted training enables zero-shot task generalization. Proceedings of the International Conference on Learning Representations 2022. Available at: https://openreview.net/forum?id=9Vrb9D0WI4.

63. Liu G, Hsu TMH, McDermott M, et al. Clinically accurate chest x-ray report generation. In: machine Learning for Healthcare Conference. PMLR 2019;106: 249–69.

64. Alfarghaly O, Khaled R, Elkorany A, et al. Automated radiology report generation using conditioned transformers. Inform Med Unlocked 2021;24:100557.

65. Pivovarov R, Elhadad N. Automated methods for the summarization of electronic health records. J Am Med Inform Assoc 2015;22(5):938–47.

66. Liang J, Tsou CH, Poddar A. A novel system for extractive clinical note summarization using EHR data. In: Proceedings of the 2nd Clinical Natural Language Processing Workshop. ; 2019:46–54.

67. Abacha AB, M'rabet Y, Zhang Y, Shivade C, Langlotz C, Demner-Fushman D. Overview of the mediqa 2021 shared task on summarization in the medical domain. In: Proceedings of the 20th Workshop on Biomedical Language Processing. ; 2021:74–85.

68. Pampari A, Raghavan P, Liang J, et al. emrqa: a large corpus for question answering on electronic medical records. Proceedings of the 2018 Conference on Empirical Methods in Natural Language Processing 2018;D18-1258:2357–68.

69. Weng WH, Chung YA, Szolovits P. Unsupervised clinical language translation. In: Proceedings of the 25th ACM SIGKDD International Conference on Knowledge Discovery & Data Mining. ; 2019:3121–3131.

70. Weizenbaum J. ELIZA—a computer program for the study of natural language communication between man and machine. Commun ACM 1966;9(1):36–45.

71. The medical futurist. The top 12 healthcare chatbots. The medical futurist. 2021. Available at: https://medicalfuturist.com/top-12-health-chatbots/. Accessed May 18, 2022.

72. Merrill MA, Althoff T. Transformer-based behavioral representation learning enables transfer learning for mobile sensing in small datasets. arXiv 2021. Available at: http://arxiv.org/abs/2107.06097.

73. Wynants L, Van Calster B, Collins GS, et al. Prediction models for diagnosis and prognosis of covid-19: systematic review and critical appraisal. BMJ 2020;369: m1328.

74. Roberts M, Driggs D, Thorpe M, et al. Common pitfalls and recommendations for using machine learning to detect and prognosticate for COVID-19 using chest radiographs and CT scans. Nat Machine Intelligence 2021;3(3):199–217.

75. Gong JJ, Naumann T, Szolovits P, Guttag JV. Predicting clinical outcomes across changing electronic health record systems. In: Proceedings of the 23rd ACM SIGKDD International Conference on Knowledge Discovery and Data Mining. ACM; 2017:1497–1505.

76. Lazer D, Kennedy R, King G, et al. The parable of google flu: traps in big data analysis. Science 2014;343(6176):1203–5.

77. Beaulieu-Jones BK, Yuan W, Brat GA, et al. Machine learning for patient risk stratification: standing on, or looking over, the shoulders of clinicians? npj Digital Med 2021;4(1):62.

78. Adam GA, Chang CHK, Haibe-Kains B, Goldenberg A. Hidden risks of machine learning applied to healthcare: unintended feedback loops between models and future data causing model degradation. In: Doshi-Velez F, Fackler J, Jung K, et al., eds Proceedings of the 5th Machine Learning for Healthcare Conference. Vol 126. Proceedings of Machine Learning Research. PMLR; 07–08 Aug 2020:710–731.

79. Subbaswamy A, Schulam P, Saria S. Preventing failures due to dataset shift: learning predictive models that transport. In: Chaudhuri K, Sugiyama M, eds Proceedings of the Twenty-Second International Conference on Artificial Intelligence and Statistics. Vol 89. Proceedings of Machine Learning Research. PMLR; 16–18 Apr 2019:3118–3127.

80. Rajkomar A, Oren E, Chen K, et al. Scalable and accurate deep learning with electronic health records. npj Digital Med 2018;1(1):18.

81. Curth A, Thoral P, van den Wildenberg W, et al. Transferring clinical prediction models across hospitals and electronic health record systems. In: Cellier P, Driessens K, editors. Machine learning and knowledge discovery in databases. Springer International Publishing; 2020. p. 605–21.

82. Oakden-Rayner L, Dunnmon J, Carneiro G, et al. Hidden stratification causes clinically meaningful failures in machine learning for medical imaging. CoRR 2019. abs/1909.12475. Available at: http://arxiv.org/abs/1909.12475.

83. Caruana R, Lou Y, Gehrke J, Koch P, Sturm M, Elhadad N. Intelligible models for healthcare: predicting pneumonia risk and hospital 30-day readmission. In: Proceedings of the 21th ACM SIGKDD International Conference on Knowledge Discovery and Data Mining. ; 2015:1721–1730.

84. Cooper GF, Abraham V, Aliferis CF, et al. Predicting dire outcomes of patients with community acquired pneumonia. J Biomed Inform 2005;38(5):347–66.

85. Zhang H, Lu AX, Abdalla M, McDermott M, Ghassemi M. Hurtful words: quantifying biases in clinical contextual word embeddings. In: Proceedings of the ACM Conference on Health, Inference, and Learning. ; 2020:110–120.

86. Pierson E, Cutler DM, Leskovec J, et al. An algorithmic approach to reducing unexplained pain disparities in underserved populations. Nat Med 2021;27(1):136–40.

87. Hall M, van der Maaten L, Gustafson L, et al. A systematic study of bias amplification. arXiv 2022;2201:11706.

88. Vyas DA, Eisenstein LG, Jones DS. Hidden in plain sight — reconsidering the use of race correction in clinical algorithms. N Engl J Med 2020;383(9):874–82.

89. McDermott MBA, Wang S, Marinsek N, et al. Reproducibility in machine learning for health research: still a ways to go. Sci Transl Med 2021;13(586):eabb1655.

90. Oala L, Murchison AG, Balachandran P, et al. Machine learning for health: algorithm auditing & quality control. J Med Syst 2021;45(12):105.

91. Vellido A. The importance of interpretability and visualization in machine learning for applications in medicine and health care. Neural Comput Appl 2020;32(24): 18069–83.
92. Yoon CH, Torrance R, Scheinerman N. Machine learning in medicine: should the pursuit of enhanced interpretability be abandoned? J Med Ethics 2021;48(9): 581–5.
93. Stiglic G, Kocbek P, Fijacko N, et al. Interpretability of machine learning-based prediction models in healthcare. Wiley Interdiscip Rev Data Min Knowl Discov 2020;10(5):e1379.
94. Jin D, Sergeeva E, Weng WH, et al. Explainable deep learning in healthcare: a methodological survey from an attribution view. Wires Mech Dis 2022;14(3): e1548.
95. Lipton ZC. The mythos of model interpretability. CoRR 2016. abs/1606.03490. Available at: http://arxiv.org/abs/1606.03490.
96. Tonekaboni S, Joshi S, McCradden MD, Goldenberg A. What clinicians want: contextualizing explainable machine learning for clinical end use. In: Doshi-Velez F, Fackler J, Jung K, et al., eds Proceedings of the 4th Machine Learning for Healthcare Conference. Vol 106. Proceedings of Machine Learning Research. PMLR; 09–10 Aug 2019:359–380.
97. Ghassemi M, Oakden-Rayner L, Beam AL. The false hope of current approaches to explainable artificial intelligence in health care. Lancet Digital Health 2021; 3(11):e745–50.
98. Poursabzi-Sangdeh F, Goldstein DG, et al. Manipulating and measuring model interpretability. In: Proceedings of the 2021 CHI Conference on Human Factors in Computing Systems. ; 2021:1–52.

Artificial Intelligence Applications in Clinical Chemistry

Dustin R. Bunch, PhD[a,b,1], Thomas JS. Durant, MD[c,1],
Joseph W. Rudolf, MD[d,e,*]

KEYWORDS

- Artificial intelligence • Machine learning • Expert systems • Clinical chemistry

KEY POINTS

- Investigation of artificial intelligence applications for the clinical chemistry laboratory has proliferated in recent years.
- Applications for artificial intelligence spanning all phases of testing (preanalytic, analytic, postanalytic) have been documented.
- Novel applications including uses in laboratory result, diagnosis, and risk prediction may transform the role of the clinical chemistry laboratory.
- Although relatively few artificial intelligence applications have been fully implemented in the clinical chemistry laboratory, the field is maturing quickly.
- Important regulatory and ethical considerations must be addressed as chemistry laboratories look to incorporate artificial intelligence technologies in routine practice.

INTRODUCTION

Investigation of artificial intelligence (AI) applications in health care has accelerated rapidly in recent years. Accordingly, there are also rapid advancements in this area applied to the clinical laboratory. In this article, advancements in AI relevant for clinical chemistry laboratories are explored.

It is important to begin with a brief classification of AI as it will be understood for the purposes of this article. AI can be classified as general (all purpose and task independent) or narrow (focused and task targeted). Although an area of active investigation,

[a] Department of Pathology and Laboratory Medicine, Nationwide Children's Hospital, 700 Children's Drive, C1923, Columbus, OH 43205-2644, USA; [b] Department of Pathology, College of Medicine, The Ohio State University, Columbus, OH 43210, USA; [c] Department of Laboratory Medicine, Yale School of Medicine, 55 Park Street, Room PS 502A, New Haven, CT 06510, USA; [d] Department of Pathology, University of Utah School of Medicine, Salt Lake City, UT 84112, USA; [e] ARUP Laboratories, 500 Chipeta Way, MC 115, Salt Lake City, UT 84108, USA
[1] Denotes co-first authors with equal contributions.
* Corresponding author.
E-mail address: joseph.rudolf@path.utah.edu

Clin Lab Med 43 (2023) 47–69
https://doi.org/10.1016/j.cll.2022.09.005
0272-2712/23/© 2022 Elsevier Inc. All rights reserved.

labmed.theclinics.com

general AI does not presently exist as defined. AI as is experienced today exists as narrow applications.

Narrow AI is a term that encompasses expert systems (ie, rules based) and machine learning (ML). Expert systems AI employs the use of rules that are explicitly programmed by a human expert (eg, defined autoverification [AV] rules). In contrast, ML-based AI achieves a similar end point but arrives there through a different approach. Relationships between narrow AI types including representative examples can be found in **Fig. 1**.

Most of the ML-enabled technology that is used in the clinical laboratory today can be classified as "supervised ML."[1] The supervision refers to there being a "ground truth" represented in the dataset.[2] An example would be a collection of digitally scanned immunofixation electrophoresis gels that are categorically labeled by a human expert as either (1) no monoclonal protein present or (2) monoclonal protein present. Using the data and the associated labels, through the process of "training," ML can find patterns within the dataset that correspond to the presence or absence of a monoclonal protein (**Fig. 2**). In contrast to expert systems, ML-based software does not require human experts to explicitly program directions to get from question to answer; however, for supervised ML, it does require human experts to explicitly define the ground truth categories, or patterns, that can be found within the dataset. In contrast, unsupervised ML relies on only the data, and does not require explicit rules or labels to find patterns in the data.

In this article, the AI applications relevant for the clinical chemistry laboratory framed through the context of the phases of testing (preanalytic, analytic, and postanalytic) are addressed. Representative examples of use cases for the sections are found in **Table 1**. Future and ethical considerations are also addressed. In select cases, the authors briefly allude to chemistry-adjacent disciplines including hematology and microbiology; however, the majority of the text is dedicated to applications within the clinical chemistry field.

PREANALYTIC

The preanalytic phase of laboratory testing involves a heterogeneous series of activities from laboratory test ordering to patient collection to specimen preparation for

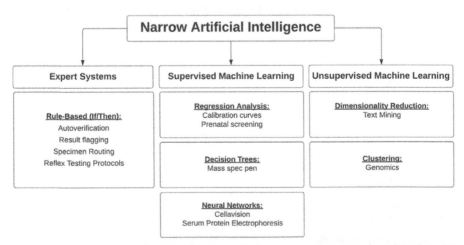

Fig. 1. Types of narrow artificial intelligence including expert systems and machine learning with representative applications.

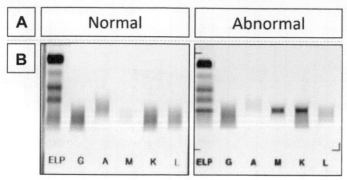

Fig. 2. Example of data that can be used for training a supervised machine learning algorithm. (*A*) Output data (label); (*B*) input data (features).

analysis[3,4] (**Fig. 3**). Some of these activities may occur with direct laboratory oversight including certain phlebotomy workflows and specimen preparation, but many occur outside the view of the laboratory. Errors in the phase of testing are unfortunately very common and have been reported to account for the majority of errors in the total testing cycle, exceeding analytic and postanalytic error rates.[5] Preanalytic errors include but are not limited to suboptimal patient preparation, labeling errors, incorrect collection containers, routing errors, and incorrect specimen preparation. Owing to their frequency and impact, the detection of preanalytic error is crucial for laboratory quality. However, these errors remain difficult to detect. Traditional approaches have included strategies such as single analyte delta checks and specimen inspection for common interferences attributable to collection (ie, hemolysis). AI applications represent an important opportunity for enhanced preanalytic error detection; this is an area of active investigation in the AI community, and recent important examples are discussed in the following sections.

Wrong Blood in Tube Detection

One important and impactful preanalytic error type is wrong blood in tube (WBIT). WBIT errors occur when a patient specimen is labeled with a patient identifier label for a different patient. WBIT errors are difficult to identify and have been shown to occur with a frequency between 0.5% and 1%.[6] Undetected, these errors lead to laboratory results being posted to the incorrect patient chart. Historically, hospital laboratories have used single-analyte delta checks where a result is compared with a previously reported value for a patient and discrepancies are investigated for possible WBIT error.

In recent years, multiple ML models were developed to improve WBIT detection.[7–11] Techniques have included classification and clustering ML methods, and have evaluated a variety of tests including common chemistry and hematology analytes. The results have been impressive yielding receiver operating characteristic (ROC) areas under the curve (AUCs) exceeding 0.99 in many cases indicating that these models are both sensitive and specific for this use case.

In one study, ML models for WBIT detection were shown to exceed human performance in detecting WBIT errors.[11] In another study by the same investigator, an ML model for WBIT detection was studied in both a decision support mode (where human operators adjudicated AI predictions before result release) and an autonomous mode (where AI predictions were released unreviewed). Interestingly, human adjudication of

Table 1
Selected representative examples for artificial intelligence in the clinical chemistry laboratory including input data, output data, artificial intelligence model, and clinical use case

Area	Input Data (Features)	Output Data (Label)	Model	Use Case
Preanalytic				
Wrong blood in tube detection[11]	Common laboratory tests including electrolytes, urea, creatinine	Presence or absence of wrong blood in tube	Neural network (also regression, classification, and ensemble)	Detect cases of wrong blood in tube
Spurious result detection[12]	Glucose and anion gap results	Presence or absence of spurious glucose result	Classification (decision tree)	Detect spurious blood glucose results
Specimen quality[17]	Coagulation test results	Presence or absence of clot in specimen	Neural network	Detect clotted specimens
Analytic				
Quality control[23]	Common chemistry results, day/time of result, predicted test result	Probability of error	Classification (logistic regression)	Detect out of control states
Result prediction/imputation[26]	18 laboratory test using patients' vitals, age, sex, and admission diagnosis	Normal or abnormal result	Ensemble (fuzzy model, logistic regression, random forest, gradient boosted trees)	Determine pretest probability of a laboratory test
Diagnosis and risk prediction[49]	Laboratory test results including complete blood cell count and comprehensive chemistry panel	Objective remission, noncompliance, or shunting	Ensemble (random forest)	Monitor thiopurine therapy
Image analysis (serum quality analysis)[15]	Images of centrifuged sample tubes	Presence or absence of interferent (eg, "hemolysis," "icterus,", or "lipemia")	Inception-Resnet-V2	Image-based system to reduce HIL test volume

Interpretation support (electrophoresis)[70]	Serum protein electrophoresis densitogram	Interpretation classification	Deep neural network	Provide possible interpretations based on data
Interpretation support (mass spectrometry)[74]	Digital chromatogram	Peak and integration parameters	Ensemble (custom tree based ML, RF, SVM, XGBtree)	Data preprocessing
Interpretation support (toxicology)[79]	Mycophenolic concentrations	0–12 hour area under the curve	XGB	Mycophenolic exposure
Postanalytic				
Autoverification[83]	13 test results, 7 delta values, age, HIL index	Automatically report or hold	Artificial neural network	Determine if a clinical result can be released
Reference intervals[88]	Numeric test results and ICD9 code	Reference interval	Multilayer feedforward artificial neural network	Reference interval determination

Abbreviations: HIL, hemolysis-icterus-lipemia; ICD9, International Classification of Diseases, Ninth Revision; RF, random forest; SVM, support vector machine.

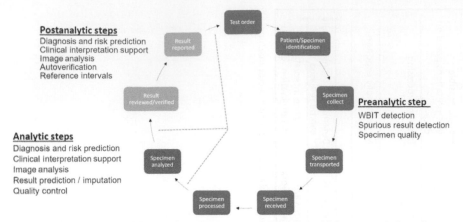

Fig. 3. Representation of the total testing process in the clinical laboratory. Below the analytic steps are common issues and/or problems in the laboratory that have a machine learning solution described in this review.

results before release was found to decrease overall performance and the investigators proposed models for WBIT detection may be best deployed in an autonomous configuration.

Given the potential for significant adverse patient outcomes, these models represent an important opportunity for preanalytic error detection. Current laboratory information system (LIS) limitations represent barriers to more complex model implementations; however, the performance of simple models (ie, decision trees) that could be supported in these legacy systems represents significant improvements over existing error detection strategies.[11]

Spurious Result Detection

Another promising area for preanalytic error detection leveraging AI applications is that of spurious result detection. Spurious results arise when a falsely elevated or decreased measurement is observed as a function of an external factor such as specimen contamination with an interfering substance. Such results can cause a treating team to conclude that a patient is experiencing a disease state that is in fact not present. A few select studies highlight the role that AI may play in detecting these events.

In one early study from 2012, the investigators developed a decision tree model to identify spurious glucose measurements resulting from specimen contamination with intravenous (IV) fluid containing glucose.[12] This type of error occurs when a specimen is incorrectly drawn off an indwelling patient line containing IV fluid or drawn from a peripheral site near the administration of IV fluid. The resulting glucose value may be significantly increased and cause the treating team to conclude the patient is experiencing significant hyperglycemia when the patient may in fact have normal glucose levels. Using a limited set of features including other common concurrent laboratory results and historical glucose values, the investigators constructed models with reasonable sensitivity (74%) and high specificity (100%) in cases in which the glucose measurement exceeded 800 mg/dL.[12]

The presence of hemolysis can also result in spurious results. For example, the lysis of red blood cells can increase the potassium present in a specimen, resulting in pseudo-hyperkalemia. In central laboratories, this phenomenon can be detected through the spectrophotometric measurement of hemolysis indices. However, this evaluation is not performed at the point of care (POC) and leaves POC laboratory methods susceptible to spurious potassium results attributable to hemolysis; this was investigated recently by a team who developed a logistic regression ML model for hemolysis prediction in POC specimens. The model was highly performant with an ROC exceeding 0.99.[13] The investigators proposed 2 possible applications for this model: retrospective quality control (QC) analysis for hemolysis rates and prospective use to identify hemolysis with specimen reflex to a central method where hemolysis could be verified.[13]

In addition to common chemistry analytes, hematology testing may also be prone to spurious results. For example, certain clinical conditions such as liver disease or the presence of abnormal hemoglobin variants may result in red cells being resistant to lysis during analysis.[14] As a result, intact red cells may be misclassified as lymphocytes leading to spurious white blood cell differentials.[14] Current analyzers are not able to detect this type of event. Accordingly, one group endeavored to develop a support vector machine (SVM) ML model to detect this condition. Using cell population data, the team was able to develop a model with accuracies of ~89% in patients with liver disease and ~98% in patients with anemia causing lysis resistance.[14]

Specimen Quality

Specimen quality is frequently evaluated in the clinical laboratory for potential impacts on analysis. In addition to the evaluation of hemolysis discussed earlier, the presence of bilirubin (icterus) and lipids (lipemia) is also frequently evaluated by spectrophotometry on automated chemistry platforms to obtain hemolysis-icterus-lipemia (HIL) indices. In other settings specimens are visually inspected and compared with job aids with pictures containing known concentrations of these substances to semiquantitatively assess the presence of HIL.

The presence of these substances may interfere with reaction chemistry leading to falsely increased or decreased results depending on the analyte of interest and method. In vitro diagnostic device manufacturers report that the effects of these substances in assay materials and laboratories may incorporate cutoffs to prevent reporting of affected specimens or add result comments noting limitations in the measurement of affected specimens.

Evaluation of specimens for HIL has limitations. In the case of visual inspection, interindividual variation in assessment is a concern.[15] Automated HIL indices may reduce variation but incur the cost of additional analysis time.[15] To improve on existing HIL assessment strategies, one group developed a convolutional neural network ML model to predict HIL based on tube images. The investigators subsequently developed a workflow in which samples likely to be affected by HIL or obstructed by the presence of a label were reflexed for HIL indices, whereas specimens unlikely to be affected had results released without automated indices.[15] This model achieved ROC exceeding 0.9.[15] Other investigators have developed ML models specific for hemolysis.[16] Additional discussion of AI imaging applications follows in the Image Analysis section.

Specimen clots may also impact specimen quality and suitability for analysis; this may be especially relevant in routine coagulation testing including such tests as prothrombin time, activated partial thromboplastin time, fibrinogen, thrombin time, and d-dimer.[17] Traditional methods for detecting clots in the laboratory include placing a wooden stick in the specimen to remove clots or inverting the tube to visually inspect the specimen.[17] These evaluations may fail to detect small clots and present occupational exposure hazards to staff.[17] To address this laboratory challenge, one group developed neural network models to identify the presence of clot in specimens ordered for common coagulation tests. The models were highly performant with ROC exceeding 0.96.

Analytic

The analytical phase of testing includes the steps of analysis of the specimen and ends with the generation of a patient result or interpretive report (see **Fig. 3**). Many studies have been performed in recent years to apply AI to the analytic phase. In this section novel AI applications are discussed including for result, diagnosis, and risk prediction as well as interpretive report generation. QC and image analysis are also addressed.

Quality Control

QC activities are fundamental components of a laboratory's quality program. Traditional clinical laboratory QC practices involve measuring liquid QC materials and evaluating the results against the known concentrations of the materials on a set schedule. Assays are determined to be in or out of control based on statistical evaluation of the data. The criteria governing this statistical control process are generally expert rules-based systems.

Although traditional liquid QC activities have significantly benefited laboratory quality over many decades, there are limitations. One significant limitation is that liquid QC provides insight into an assay's control only at the time that it is performed, often once every 24 hours. As a result, laboratories have limited insight into an assay's performance between liquid QC events.

To address this gap, multiple investigators and groups have been actively developing and refining the concept of patient-based real-time QC (PBRTQC).[18–22] In PBRTQC, patient results are treated as continuous QC material and algorithms are developed to identify changes in assay performance in real time. Simple models incorporate averages of blocks of patient results. As error is introduced to the assay system, the average will change. When identified control limits are exceeded a user is notified. More sophisticated models may include data transformation and weighting algorithms. Simulation has been used to systematically optimize configuration including truncation limits and optimize block sizes.[18] Although modeling and simulation are leveraged in the development of these QC tools, the model itself remains a rules-based system.

ML applications for QC are more nascent but have promise. For example, in one study, a multianalyte logistic regression model was developed for a common chemistry panel including 14 analytes.[23] For each analyte, the value was predicted based on the remaining analytes in the panel and compared with the measured value.[23] Probability of the presence of error was predicted based on differences between the predicted and measured results.[23]

In another study, a group developed an R programming language package including a supervised ML model to assess mass spectrometry (MS) peak quality due to poor chromatography or interference.[24] Following training by a user, the model can be applied to large data sets to quickly identify peaks of poor quality.[24] In a separate study, a team developed a support vector regression model coupled to QC samples to address intrabatch effects in a MS application.[25]

These examples hint at the promise of ML for QC. Although current examples are limited in the literature, additional AI applications for QC are sure to emerge in the coming years.

Result Prediction and Imputation

As applied to the clinical laboratory, imputation is the ability to predict a patient's laboratory results from clinical information available in the electronic health record (EHR) or LIS, which can include diagnosis, vitals, previous laboratory results, imagining, and other available information. The utility of imputation includes determining pretest probability of a specific laboratory test, determining if a marker is redundant, calculating the result of an unordered test, and filling in missing data elements required to process a patient through the ML system.

Using ML to determine pretest probability may allow clinicians to identify low-yield tests in specific departments at the time of order and prevent them from ordering. The Valderrama and colleagues[26] study is an example of pretest probability imputation, which included 48,672 patients in the intensive care unit from Alberta, Canada. The comparison method was based on conditional entropy and conditional probability. The first ML algorithm performed predictions of normal patient results for 18 laboratory test using patients' vitals, age, sex, and admission diagnosis features. A second ML algorithm performed predictions for abnormal patient results using the same 18 tests using the data from algorithm 1 and entropy and pretest probability features. An ensemble ML model was created combining fuzzy model, logistic regression, random forest (RF), and gradient boosted trees and optimized using 10 parameters (specificity, sensitivity, accuracy, precision, negative predictive value, F1 score, area under the ROC, area under the precision-recall curve, mean G, and index balanced accuracy). The outcome of this study indicated that the combined features performed better than the individual features. These types of tools may allow for the identification of low-yield testing and could help conserve patient blood for those in the intensive care unit. With pretest probability being one of the major features, this type of ML could be best suited for long-term in-patients where there are multiple tests performed in a short period.

Another useful function of imputation concerns identifying laboratory tests that may be redundant and/or unordered. Redundant laboratory tests can increase turnaround times and increase the likelihood of a false-positive. Laboratory testing, especially in the chemistry section, often uses a population-derived central 95% for reference intervals (RI). From a statistical perspective, for every 20 tests ordered, one of those tests would be a false-positive based solely on the definition used in the creation of the RI. Three recent examples of imputation for this purpose are Lidbury and colleagues,[27] Luo and colleagues,[28] and Kurstjens and colleagues.[29]

The Lidbury study identified the liver function test, alkaline phosphatase and alanine aminotransaminase as strong correlates of γ-glutamyl transferase (GGT) and then attempted to predict the GGT using an SVM model. Results from 25,420 patients were used with a 70:30 train:test split with 10-fold training and testing cross-validation. The decision tree yielded an accuracy of 83.9% for the GGT normal range and 92.6% for the elevated range, whereas the SVM had a prediction accuracy of 78.2% and 79% for the normal and elevated ranges, respectively. The Luo and Kurstjens studies both used imputation of ferritin for a proof-of-principle study. Ferritin, a marker for iron deficiency, is not routinely ordered, whereas a complete blood cell count is routinely ordered. The Luo study used 42 analytes to predict the ferritin result. However, many of the 42 analytes had missing data (14%–65%); before it could be used for the prediction of ferritin it had to be complete, which was accomplished through 4 imputation methods (mean, multiple imputation with chained equations-full [MICE-full], multiple imputation with chained equations-select [MICE-sel], and missForest). Next regression was used to predict a numeric value for ferritin using linear regression, Bayesian linear regression, random forest regression (RFR), and lasso regression (lasso). Finally, a classifier was used to determine the normal or elevated range for ferritin using logistic regression with the area under the receiver operator curve as the optimization parameter. In addition, a univariate analysis was performed to determine the contribution of each test to the ferritin prediction. missForest was identified as the best algorithm for imputation of missing results for ferritin classification ROC of 0.964. The assays that contributed most to the ferritin classification were mean corpuscular hemoglobin (MCH), mean corpuscular volume (MCV), and Total iron binding capacity (TIBC) with AUC of 0.84, 0.83, and 0.85, respectively. The Kurstjens study found that MCH, MCV, age, and C-Reactive protein (CRP) were the best predictors for ferritin. Kurstjens and colleagues[29] also placed the ML algorithm in clinical use for 21 work days and were able to identify 18 new iron deficiencies. As with the WBIT algorithm, the investigators found an automated method was more accurate than either the specialist and a specialist-ML combination.

As seen in the aforementioned example, ML is sensitive to missing data and can give erroneous results if missing data are present or ML calculations are unable to be performed. This is a common issue that can compromise the function of an ML pipeline because ML algorithms often require a complete data set to perform the ML prediction. Real patients often have missing data that is required by the ML algorithm. To include these patients in the ML pipelines, the missing data need to be supplied. Common imputation methods for missing data include those previously described (mean, MICE-full, MICE-sel, and missForest), but these techniques are not suited for temporal imputation. Luo and colleagues[30] describe a method to do temporal imputation called 3D multiple imputation with chained equations or 3D-MICE. Normalized root-mean-square (NRMS) error determines the difference between results with a smaller value indicating better performance of the imputation methods. Thirteen common clinical laboratory tests for 3,130,501 test results were compared with MICE (NRMS 0.373), Gaussian process (0.358), and 3D-MICE (0.342) indicating 3D-MICE was the better temporal imputation method.

In addition to imputation of unordered test results, imputation can also be used to identify testing that is no longer useful and could be removed from a test menu. If a test can be accurately determined from other test results, it would indicate that the test in question is redundant. Because the test is redundant in light of other tests, it may be better to substitute a calculation for a measured result or to stop relying on the test in clinical settings. The laboratory has created many new and useful tests in the last 100 years, but it can be challenging to remove tests even when new tests are better suited to answer the clinical question.

Diagnosis and Risk Prediction

AI applications present a unique opportunity to improve over existing methods for diagnosis and risk prediction based on clinical laboratory data. Significant progress has occurred in recent years to develop AI models for a variety of disease states based on either laboratory data alone or in conjunction with other patient data such as demographics or other clinical findings. A representative sample of these applications with a focus on those emphasizing chemistry data are discussed in this section.

Early AI applications in this area focused on risk-based models for common clinical conditions. For example, multiple regression-based models incorporating laboratory biomarkers and limited clinical data were developed to aid in predicting the risk of identifying prostate cancer at biopsy in patients with nonconclusive total prostate-specific antigen results.[31–33] Risk scores derived from these models can be used to further stratify patient risk and inform the decision to proceed to prostate biopsy, reducing the risk of unnecessary biopsy in some patients.

Noninvasive risk prediction models have also been developed for use in identifying patients with nonalcoholic steatohepatitis (NASH), a subset of nonalcoholic fatty liver disease.[34,35] Patients with NASH have heightened risk of developing complications such as cirrhosis and carcinoma.[35] Fibrosis staging was historically performed by liver biopsy.[34,35] Multiple groups have developed noninvasive AI models using biochemical data augmented by patient data, and in some cases imaging findings, to stratify patients at risk for further progression.[34,35]

Similar approaches incorporating specialized biomarkers have been leveraged to develop models to predict decline in kidney function in patients with type 2 diabetes.[36,37] The developers of these models propose that risk stratification may facilitate early intervention to prevent further progression.[37]

One potential limitation to some of the models described earlier is the proprietary nature of either the model calculation and/or incorporated biomarkers; this may limit the ability of others in the field to interrogate the models. It may also limit which laboratories are able to perform the testing and interpretation. It remains to be seen what effect the proliferation of proprietary scoring models has on the diagnostics market including costs and availability for patients.

Risk scores have also been applied in the acute care setting to predict a wide variety of clinical outcomes including the development of iatrogenic hypoglycemia, acute kidney injury, and intensive care unit mortality.[38–41] Prediction of these event types may allow for early intervention, decreasing morbidity and mortality. In some cases, the models rely heavily on EHR data to identify features. Owing to the heterogeneity of data structure and storage in the EHR, model interoperability between institutions may be more challenging than models relying on laboratory data alone or those incorporating limited demographic data.

AI applications have also shown promise for diagnosis within the clinical laboratory using laboratory data alone. For example, models have been developed to assist with evaluation of highly complex laboratory data, such as in the cases of MS data for steroid profiles and plasma amino acid profiles.[42–44] ML models developed for these settings have been shown to differentiate abnormal from normal profiles, and even make diagnosis predictions.[42–44] Classification models such as these may reduce subjectivity in interpretation and increase availability to laboratories with less specialist expertise.[42,43]

Another interesting diagnostic application for AI is the differentiation of clinical conditions with overlapping laboratory findings. For example, iron deficiency anemia and thalassemia trait may both present as hypochromic microcytic anemia and may be difficult to differentiate based on existing red blood cell profile cutoffs. This presents a significant diagnostic challenge in regions where thalassemia trait is common. In one such region (Thailand), researchers developed an automated prediction model based on cell profile data to discriminate iron deficiency anemia from thalassemia trait.[45] This model was published as a Web-based application to assist in differentiating these conditions.[45] Users simply enter common laboratory values and are presented with a risk prediction for thalassemia trait versus iron deficiency anemia.[45]

AI leveraging predominantly laboratory data has also been used to predict treatment appropriateness and response. Some notable examples have addressed prediction of antibiotic susceptibility in the microbiology laboratory.[46–48] Specific to the chemistry laboratory, one group developed a model to predict therapeutic response in patients receiving thiopurine treatment of inflammatory bowel disease.[49] Monitoring patients on thiopurine therapy is crucial due to the narrow therapeutic index. The tree-based model incorporates common clinical chemistry and hematology results to classify patients as having 1 of 3 outcomes: objective remission, nonadherence, or preferential shunting to 6-methylmercaptopurine.[49] The algorithm is offered as an assay orderable through the clinical laboratory.[49]

Image Analysis

Most workflows in today's clinical chemistry laboratory offer limited opportunities for digital imaging. However, a few tasks remain present in modern workflows that require a visual assessment by a human operator. With the increasing need to improve laboratory throughput, there is an incentive to leverage digital imaging technology to automate these tasks. Accordingly, recent efforts have evaluated the use of AI/ML in this setting to optimize workflows related to specimen processing, preanalytic error detection, and clinical decision support for assays that require visual inspection.

As laboratory technology continues to evolve and data become more accessible, there is an emerging opportunity to explore novel methods that can detect preanalytic errors that occur outside the laboratory. In 2014, Hawker and colleagues[50] described an imaging-based device that automatically detected discrepancies between the name printed on the specimen laboratory and the name linked in the LIS. Implementation of this tool found an error rate of 4.6 per 100,000 patient specimens that were not otherwise detected by preexisting quality assurance protocols. Furthermore, the study demonstrated that implementing this technology in modern automated chemistry track systems is feasible, with a per specimen processing time of approximately 3 seconds.

Although the technology described by Hawker and colleagues[50] is not widely implemented in commercially available systems today, it highlights that the modular nature of modern automated chemistry systems allows for opportunities to append imaging-based, safety-driven automation modules to existing systems. To this end, some commercially available automated chemistry systems have begun implementing similar imaging modules to evaluate other kinds of preanalytical errors.

Historically, specimen tubes were visually inspected for the presence of excessive lipemia or hemolysis before testing; however, this practice has largely been replaced by the HIL (hemolysis, icteric, and lipemic) indices, which are now commonly measured on automated chemistry instruments. Today, some platforms now offer digital imaging of samples to measure the hue of the sample to evaluate for preanalytical sources of error, such as hemolysis.[15,16] These digital imaging-based checks may complement existing methods (eg, HIL indices).

Beyond specimen processing workflows, AI/ML-enabled technologies also show promise in streamlining assays that require manual interpretation by an expert human operator. Urine test strips, often used at POC, are subject to interpretation variability, which can lead to analytic errors. Image-based automation of test strips has shown promise to reduce this variability, improve analytical sensitivity, and by deploying image recognition algorithms on smartphones, provide interpretation at the POC or at the point of testing (eg, home testing).[51–53] Urine microscopic analyzers have also seen the adoption of image-based automation that relies on pattern recognition to identify and preclassify urine particulates for expert operator review.[51,54–57] Various studies have shown a good correlation between technologies such as these and the predicate, manual microscopic method.[51,58] Similarly, there has been significant interest and progress in the area of adapting computer vision and ML to the automated analysis of digital microscopic analysis of hematology specimens.[59–61]

The diagnosis of autoimmune diseases is often aided by immunofluorescence testing that seeks to characterize antibody-binding patterns against macromolecular components of mammalian cells via microscopy.[62] However, recognition of these patterns can be time-consuming and reliant on technical expertise for accurate characterization. Accordingly, there is both academic and commercial interest in automating antinuclear antibody pattern recognition, and image-based pattern recognition is a common approach.[63] In recent years, method comparison studies have shown similar performance between automated and conventional microscopic interpretation of anti-neutrophil cytoplasmic antibody (ANCA) testing in a variety of disease types.[64,65] Although these technologies may still benefit from expert operator review, these approaches streamline sample processing and minimize interpretation variability. Recent data suggest that there may also be benefits to assisting those with limited experience interpreting ANCA-related microscopy.[66]

Last, gel electrophoresis is a commonly used method to identify paraproteins, the presence of which may aid in the diagnosis of various types of lymphoproliferative disorders or monoclonal gammopathies (eg, Waldenström macroglobulinemia or multiple myeloma) (see **Fig. 2**). The interpretation of gel electrophoresis, similar to assays previously described, is a manually intensive and time-consuming process that is subject to intraindividual and interindividual bias. Accordingly, recent literature has evaluated AI/ML-based detection of paraproteins from images of digitally scanned electrophoresis gels.[67–69] Although this approach is not widely commercialized, initial results are promising and may serve as a tool that can assist laboratories that are more comfortable with gel-based paraprotein detection and streamline test throughput to meet growing demands for testing.

Report Interpretation and Generation (Clinical Interpretation Support)

Electrophoresis
Serum protein electrophoresis (SPEP) is a critical test for multiple myeloma and useful for gross disorders of serum proteins. The primary clinical indication of the test is to identify and manage patients with multiple myeloma. The method is able to detect the most abundant serum proteins (albumin, immunoglobulins, therapeutic monoclonal antibodies, and others). Patient samples are loaded onto gel separation cartridges where a charge and solvent are applied; this causes the proteins to separate, and when dye is added creates bands that can be digitized using a densitometer and translated into a chromatogram and numeric results. The interpretation of SPEPs requires extensive training, which includes a keen eye and expert pattern matching to identify all possible variations. ML could be a valuable tool to improve interpretations and possibly allow for AV in the future. A recent study by Chabrun and colleagues[70] demonstrates that an effective tool can be created to support clinical interpretation of SPEP results. SPECTR (serum protein electrophoresis computer-assisted recognition) applied a deep neural network to achieve an Area Under Curve Receiver Operator Characteristic (AUC-ROC) of 0.99 for M-spikes. In addition, the application was packaged so other laboratories could implement it at their institutions.

Mass spectrometry
MS in the clinical laboratory is a broad topic. This section focuses on small-molecule liquid chromatography tandem mass spectrometry (LC-MS/MS). There are other interesting applications including intraoperative or microbial MS if further study is of interest to the reader.[71,72]

LC-MS/MS is the most prevalent LC-MS system in use within clinical laboratories at this time. In many laboratories, LC-MS/MS data review is managed with an expert system rule engine or manual review using expert-based rules. At present, there is one commercial software available (ASCENT by Indigo BioAutomation) that does peak isolation and evaluation using complex rules or ML and manages calibration and QC review.[73] However, this is a closed system without publications concerning the ML in use. Recently, an R package was published that uses ML for data preprocessing and ML-based quality review using r 11-nor-9-carboxy-delta9-

tetrahydrocannabinol (THC-COOH) as a test case of how ML improves turn around time (TAT) and productivity by reducing the manual data review required.[74,75] Owing to technology involved in LC-MS/MS, a multianalyte panel is often performed. As an example, a drug of abuse panel may have 5 and up to 150 analytes in some newer drug panels. A typical LC-MS/MS batch requires review of the calibrations and QC for each analyte, followed by review of the peaks for shape, quality, tailing, and retention time. Using ML algorithms like those in Eilertz and Yu for an LC-MS/MS pipeline could greatly reduce the fatigue laboratory scientist experience and may improve accuracy, TAT, and overall quality.

The application of ML for interpretation of LC-MS/MS data especially in newborn screening (NBS), where complex panels are used and multiple panels may need to be synthesized, is experiencing a rapid expansion, at least on the research level. Examples of this recent work includes using random forest (RF) to reduce false-positive in MS/MS NBS, a custom tree-based ML for the differential diagnosis of peroxisomal disorders, and an ensemble of RF, extreame gradient boosting trees (XGBT), and weighted-subspace RF was able to predict the interpretation of plasma amino acids.[43,76,77] Although these are promising, they likely require clinical validation and additional data before clinicians will be comfortable using these ML due to the importance of the interpretation.

Toxicology

Clinical toxicology can be separated into many subspecialties. One subspecialty that is well-positioned for ML is therapeutic drug monitoring (TDM), which is used to manage adverse effects from drugs that typically have narrow therapeutic effects and variable individual metabolism such as immunosuppressants. Patients with TDM are under managed care with a known drug and have routine blood tests to monitor drug levels. The extensive data these consecutive blood tests generate improve the feasibility of developing ML algorithms to predict future dose responses. TDM ML can be applied for various reasons including to reduce the amount of blood sampling required to manage treatment, to predict an optimal dose of the drug, and to identify changes in metabolism that may be an early indicator of the clinical course for the patient. Recent examples of ML deployed to address these issues can be found in the study by Labriffe and colleagues,[78] which focuses on reduced sampling, from the same group Woillard and colleagues[79] who used ML to predict the optimal dose for mycophenolic acid (a compound that has been difficult to predict with traditional methods), and from Burghelea and colleagues[80] in which the investigators were able to identify tacrolimus toxicity without performing a biopsy (the current gold standard).[78–80]

Another area of clinical toxicology is acute toxicology where a substance (illicit, prescribed, and/or environmental) is ingested. These patients often present in the emergency department, and the ingested substance may or may not be known. These situations rely heavily on the experience and familiarity of the clinical toxicologist to quickly and accurately diagnose and treat the condition. Many toxic substances are time and concentration dependent so the quicker an antidote or counteracting drug is administered, the better the outcome for the patient. Toxic substances often have similar nonspecific symptoms, which make diagnosis and treatment more difficult. Chary and colleagues[81] have demonstrated an ML tool that could be an aid to diagnosis allowing for improved speed of diagnosis and subsequently treatment. Although the algorithm is a proof of concept, the ML used probabilistic logic networks to achieve levels equivalent to experts while allowing for an explainable algorithm.

POSTANALYTIC

The postanalytic phase of the laboratory testing process deals with the reporting of the data from instruments into the LIS and subsequently the EHR (see **Fig. 3**). AV and RI reflect the reporting of results and interpretation of results, respectively.

Autoverification

AV is a process with 2 purposes (1) to identify patient samples that require a higher level of intervention from a clinical laboratory scientist and (2) to release routine patient samples that do not require intervention. Typically, AV systems are built on a curated, expert rules system. Advantages of AV systems include the application of a common set of criteria for all samples and users and improvement of error detection over a manual rule criteria system.[82] The major disadvantage to this type of system is the requirement of an expert curator with limited resources (ie, published literature, consultation with colleagues, and individual experience). ML is a tool to complement the expert and allow for relationships to be derived that exist within the LIS or EHR data, but escaped the notice of expert curators.

A 2016 publication demonstrates an artificial neural network (ANN) for the total replacement of the traditional rule-based AV systems. The study by Demirci and colleagues[83] used 252,847 samples collected over a 1-year period, which was reduced to 152,226 samples after exclusion criteria were applied such as samples with zero, negative, or nonnumeric values. The algorithm was created using Weka Software, which turned the predictive value into a cutoff point that yielded accept, reject, and intermediate with further investigation of the intermediate. The ANN was compared against a panel of specialists with a consensus of 7 of 8 specialists required; this seems to have been a proof of principle because there was no mention of integration into the clinical workflow.

Wang and colleagues[84] published a hybrid system with red-flag rejection rules supplemented with an ML architecture using an ensemble of the top-three models (Naïve Bayes, K-Nearest Neighbor, Random Forest, Xgboost) with the top three models not indicated in the publication. The original optimization was performed using the classic AUC, while the results were satisfactory pass rate of 92.13% and false-negative rate (FNR) of 0.67%.[84] However, they were concerned with the FNR and opted for a second round of modeling, which introduced oversampling and changed the main evaluating parameter from AUC to FNR. These changes yielded an FNR of 0.095% with a pass rate of 89.60%. Following exclusion criteria 196,591 samples were available for ML testing, which were collected from data over a 14-month period. Like the Demirici study, experts were used during the building (manually labeling) and testing of the ML model in the clinical setting. The ML system showed an improved access when compared with the predicate method especially for the in-patient population, which increased the average passing rate from 0.35% to 0.85%. In addition, the number of invalid reports (held for clinical laboratory scientist review) dropped from an average of 50 per half hour to less than 20 per half hour.

An issue raised by these studies concerned the accessibility of the data needed to build the ML models. Acquiring the accepted data from the LIS is straightforward, but rejected data are not as readily available and need to be mined from the middleware or other source. Given the clinical impact of these results and potential risks, ML models (especially nonexplainable or closed systems) are unlikely to replace current practices in the near future. However, hybrid models where ML assists during resulting and holds for further manual review may be accepted in routine practice.

Reference Intervals

Clinical laboratories are required to provide interpretative information such as RI to accompany results. For many tests in clinical chemistry, RI are the totality of interpretative information supplied. RI are typically defined as the interval that contains the central 95% of results from healthy patients. However, there are many factors that can affect the RI such as assay, population, sex, age, reproductive, and tanner stage. Historically, RI were calculated by hand or by the Hoffmann[85] or Bhattacharya[86] methods using predetermined healthy subjects. With the voluminous data from the LIS and EHR, RI can be generated by indirect methods. For a review on indirect RI see Jones and colleagues.[87] However, robust statistical methods are required to separate the normal population signal from the pathologic signal. ML is a recent addition to the previous robust statistical methods.[88,89]

The Poole article describes the creation of the Laboratory Information Mining for Individualized Thresholds (LIMIT), which is an unsupervised learning algorithm that uses outlier detection and International Classification of Diseases, Ninth Revision, codes to remove pathologic codes and perform RI for analytes. This algorithm is not a traditional ML method, but is understandable and could easily be performed manually. This algorithm yields an explainable (ie, non–black box method) ML application. The Yang article uses a multilayer feedforward ANN to incorporate geographic information (altitude, annual sunshine hours, annual average relative humidity, annual average temperature, and annual average precipitation) into RI for erythrocyte sedimentation rates (ESR). The investigators found the ANN to be more stable than linear regression models and able to work with covariate data. RI are an area of active interest and may see an increase in the application of ML in the coming years as more data scientists engage with this field.

FUTURE AND ETHICAL CONSIDERATIONS

The adoption of AI/ML-enabled technology offers both opportunity and risk. Successful integration of this technology, as defined by optimizing for the opportunity and minimizing risk, will require careful creation and adherence to the unique ethical principles that are associated with applied AI/ML. There are many reviews of AI ethics in the medical literature, and recently an excellent overview of the ethical tenets that are most relevant to the practice of pathology and laboratory medicine.[90] Some principles may be outside the scope of interest for this article; however, those relating to scientific integrity, validation, and health equity and justice are briefly discussed here. For the interested reader, further information on AI/ML ethics can be found in recent literature.[91–93]

Clinical decision support (CDS) tools are being increasingly integrated with EHRs. Some modern CDS tools use AI/ML technology and often rely on laboratory data as input for prediction algorithms.[94] The concept of laboratory data being used as input for downstream AI/ML-enabled CDS tools is both a novel consideration for laboratorians and a useful framework for discussing the ethics associated with validating ML models that are deployed in production environments. Today, when clinical laboratories change a test method or calculation (eg, fourth- to fifth-generation troponin, implementation of new estimated glomerular filtration equation), there are often locations in the downstream EHR system that need to be updated to account for that change. Some examples include order preference lists, clinical guidance pop-ups, and shortcuts used during note writing.

For health care institutions that have implemented ML-enabled CDS, this would require a new kind of update wherein test result mappings need to be updated for

CDS-model input data. In addition, whether there is a need to revalidate CDS model performance remains an open question with such a change. This is particularly relevant for laboratory test changes that alter the distribution of result values for a local population, because these changes may influence the performance of downstream ML applications. Going forward, it remains to be seen to what degree laboratorians can and should be aware of downstream applications that take laboratory data as input, and the level of their involvement in their implementation and revalidation or reverification.

The evolving regulatory landscape may partly influence laboratorian involvement with the implementation and monitoring of ML-enabled software. The US Food and Drug Administration has released draft documents outlining the proposed regulatory structure for AI/ML-enabled software as a medical device (SaMD) and Good Machine Learning Practices.[95] These documents introduce the concept of a "predetermined change control plan," which would allow manufacturers to specify what part of their software they plan to update (ie, retrain/tune) and the protocol for effectuating changes; this would allow manufacturers to leverage the adaptive nature of ML without requiring resubmission when model weights are updated. However, it remains unclear who will take responsibility for revalidation or reverification requirements, if those are put in place, and whether these changes will require effort from the health care institution, manufacturer, or both. Furthermore, how these regulations may be integrated into existing laboratory regulation frameworks (eg, CAP/CLIA and state DPH) or proposed legislation for laboratory developed tests remains an evolving area of discussion.

Patient safety is a close corollary to model validation that can be viewed through the lens of evidence-based medicine, a longstanding framework used to guide judicious clinical decision making in a way that optimizes the benefit-to-risk ratio for patients. A recent publication by Wilson and colleagues[96] describes a double-blinded, multicenter, parallel, randomized controlled trial that sought to determine if AI-based electronic alerts (e-alerts) for acute kidney injury (AKI) improved patient outcomes. The findings were that the alerts did not reduce the risk of the primary outcome measure and found that alerts were associated with a higher risk of death at 14 days in nonteaching hospitals.[96] In addition, a recent systematic review of randomized AKI e-alert trials pooled data from 6 studies and found no associated reductions in mortality (odds ratio [OR], 1.05; 95% confidence interval [CI], 0.84–1.31), the need for renal replacement therapy (OR, 1.20; 95% CI, 0.91–1.57), or change in the use of fluid therapy (OR, 2.18; 95% CI, 0.46–10.31).[97]

Last, as consensus is reached on the benefit-to-risk ratio for a given intervention or practice, health equity states that both the benefit and the risk should be distributed equally among community members. Historically, the medical field has implemented practices that have disadvantaged members of minority communities. A prominent example in the field of clinical chemistry is the use of race-based equations for estimated glomerular filtration rate. At present, there is growing concern that the AI-ML-enabled software may similarly perpetuate population-level disparities.[98] As we look ahead to the development, implementation, and clinical use of AI/ML algorithms, further research is needed to elucidate a better path toward an equitable adoption of these novel technologies.

SUMMARY

As we have seen in this article, significant strides have been made in the development of AI applications in the clinical chemistry laboratory in recent years, and we expect this trend to accelerate further. The applications have profound implications for the practice of clinical chemistry spanning all phases of testing. Although there have been relatively few applications fully implemented for clinical use, the authors envision that these workflows are imminent. Important regulatory and ethical considerations will need to be addressed. However, the authors expect AI applications to fundamentally transform clinical chemistry and usher in a new era of efficient and effective health care.

DISCLOSURE

All authors report no relevant disclosures for this work.

REFERENCES

1. Herman DS, Rhoads DD, Schulz WL, et al. Artificial intelligence and mapping a new direction in laboratory medicine: a review. Clin Chem 2021;67(11):1466–82.
2. Smith KP, Wang H, Durant TJS, et al. Applications of artificial intelligence in clinical microbiology testing. Clin Microbiol Newsl 2020;42(8):61–70.
3. Lima-Oliveira G, Volanski W, Lippi G, et al. Pre-analytical phase management: a review of the procedures from patient preparation to laboratory analysis. Scand J Clin Lab Invest 2017;77(3):153–63.
4. Alavi N, Khan SH, Saadia A, et al. Challenges in preanalytical phase of laboratory medicine: rate of blood sample nonconformity in a tertiary care hospital. EJIFCC 2020;31(1):21–7.
5. Carraro P, Plebani M. Errors in a stat laboratory: types and frequencies 10 years later. Clin Chem 2007;53(7):1338–42.
6. Dzik WH, Murphy MF, Andreu G, et al. An international study of the performance of sample collection from patients. Vox Sang 2003;85(1):40–7.
7. Rosenbaum MW, Baron JM. Using machine learning-based multianalyte delta checks to detect wrong blood in tube errors. Am J Clin Pathol 2018;150(6):555–66.
8. Mitani T, Doi S, Yokota S, et al. Highly accurate and explainable detection of specimen mix-up using a machine learning model. Clin Chem Lab Med 2020;58(3):375–83.
9. Zhou R, Liang YF, Cheng HL, et al. A highly accurate delta check method using deep learning for detection of sample mix-up in the clinical laboratory. Clin Chem Lab Med 2021. https://doi.org/10.1515/cclm-2021-1171.
10. Farrell CL. Decision support or autonomous artificial intelligence? The case of wrong blood in tube errors. Clin Chem Lab Med 2021. https://doi.org/10.1515/cclm-2021-0873.
11. Farrell CJ. Identifying mislabelled samples: machine learning models exceed human performance. Ann Clin Biochem 2021;58(6):650–2.
12. Baron JM, Mermel CH, Lewandrowski KB, et al. Detection of preanalytic laboratory testing errors using a statistically guided protocol. Am J Clin Pathol 2012;138(3):406–13.
13. Benirschke RC, Gniadek TJ. Detection of falsely elevated point-of-care potassium results due to hemolysis using predictive analytics. Am J Clin Pathol 2020;154(2):242–7.
14. Bigorra L, Larriba I, Gutierrez-Gallego R. Machine learning algorithms for the detection of spurious white blood cell differentials due to erythrocyte lysis resistance. J Clin Pathol 2019;72(6):431–7.
15. Yang C, Li D, Sun D, et al. A deep learning-based system for assessment of serum quality using sample images. Clin Chim Acta 2022;531:254–60.

16. Shi X, Deng Y, Fang Y, et al. A hemolysis image detection method based on GAN-CNN-ELM. Comput Math Methods Med 2022;2022:1558607.
17. Fang K, Dong Z, Chen X, et al. Using machine learning to identify clotted specimens in coagulation testing. Clin Chem Lab Med 2021;59(7):1289–97.
18. Ng D, Polito FA, Cervinski MA. Optimization of a moving averages program using a simulated annealing algorithm: the goal is to monitor the process not the patients. Clin Chem 2016;62(10):1361–71.
19. van Rossum HH. Moving average quality control: principles, practical application and future perspectives. Clin Chem Lab Med 2019;57(6):773–82.
20. van Rossum HH, van den Broek D. Ten-month evaluation of the routine application of patient moving average for real-time quality control in a hospital setting. J Appl Lab Med 2020;5(6):1184–93.
21. Smith JD, Badrick T, Bowling F. A direct comparison of patient-based real-time quality control techniques: the importance of the analyte distribution. Ann Clin Biochem 2020;57(3):206–14.
22. Loh TP, Bietenbeck A, Cervinski MA, et al. Recommendation for performance verification of patient-based real-time quality control. Clin Chem Lab Med 2020; 58(8):1205–13.
23. Sampson ML, Gounden V, van Deventer HE, et al. CUSUM-Logistic Regression analysis for the rapid detection of errors in clinical laboratory test results. Clin Biochem 2016;49(3):201–7.
24. Toghi Eshghi S, Auger P, Mathews WR. Quality assessment and interference detection in targeted mass spectrometry data using machine learning. Clin Proteomics 2018;15:33.
25. Kuligowski J, Sanchez-Illana A, Sanjuan-Herraez D, et al. Intra-batch effect correction in liquid chromatography-mass spectrometry using quality control samples and support vector regression (QC-SVRC). Analyst 2015;140(22): 7810–7.
26. Valderrama CE, Niven DJ, Stelfox HT, et al. Predicting abnormal laboratory blood test results in the intensive care unit using novel features based on information theory and historical conditional probability: observational study. JMIR Med Inform 2022;10(6):e35250.
27. Lidbury BA, Richardson AM, Badrick T. Assessment of machine-learning techniques on large pathology data sets to address assay redundancy in routine liver function test profiles. Diagnosis (Berl) 2015;2(1):41–51.
28. Luo Y, Szolovits P, Dighe AS, et al. Using machine learning to predict laboratory test results. Am J Clin Pathol 2016;145(6):778–88.
29. Kurstjens S, de Bel T, van der Horst A, et al. Automated prediction of low ferritin concentrations using a machine learning algorithm. Clin Chem Lab Med 2022. https://doi.org/10.1515/cclm-2021-1194.
30. Luo Y, Szolovits P, Dighe AS, et al. 3D-MICE: integration of cross-sectional and longitudinal imputation for multi-analyte longitudinal clinical data. J Am Med Inform Assoc 2018;25(6):645–53.
31. Duffy MJ. Biomarkers for prostate cancer: prostate-specific antigen and beyond. Clin Chem Lab Med 2020;58(3):326–39.
32. Catalona WJ, Partin AW, Sanda MG, et al. A multicenter study of [-2]pro-prostate specific antigen combined with prostate specific antigen and free prostate specific antigen for prostate cancer detection in the 2.0 to 10.0 ng/ml prostate specific antigen range. J Urol 2011;185(5):1650–5.

33. Parekh DJ, Punnen S, Sjoberg DD, et al. A multi-institutional prospective trial in the USA confirms that the 4Kscore accurately identifies men with high-grade prostate cancer. Eur Urol 2015;68(3):464–70.

34. Yilmaz Y, Eren F. Identification of a support vector machine-based biomarker panel with high sensitivity and specificity for nonalcoholic steatohepatitis. Clin Chim Acta 2012;414:154–7.

35. Woreta TA, Van Natta ML, Lazo M, et al. Validation of the accuracy of the FAST score for detecting patients with at-risk nonalcoholic steatohepatitis (NASH) in a North American cohort and comparison to other non-invasive algorithms. PLoS One 2022;17(4):e0266859.

36. Chan L, Nadkarni GN, Fleming F, et al. Derivation and validation of a machine learning risk score using biomarker and electronic patient data to predict progression of diabetic kidney disease. Diabetologia 2021;64(7):1504–15.

37. Connolly P, Stapleton S, Mosoyan G, et al. Analytical validation of a multi-biomarker algorithmic test for prediction of progressive kidney function decline in patients with early-stage kidney disease. Clin Proteomics 2021;18(1):26.

38. Mathioudakis NN, Abusamaan MS, Shakarchi AF, et al. Development and validation of a machine learning model to predict near-term risk of iatrogenic hypoglycemia in hospitalized patients. JAMA Netw Open 2021;4(1):e2030913.

39. Tomasev N, Glorot X, Rae JW, et al. A clinically applicable approach to continuous prediction of future acute kidney injury. Nature 2019;572(7767):116–9.

40. Chiofolo C, Chbat N, Ghosh E, et al. Automated continuous acute kidney injury prediction and surveillance: a random forest model. Mayo Clin Proc 2019; 94(5):783–92.

41. Anand RS, Stey P, Jain S, et al. Predicting mortality in diabetic ICU patients using machine learning and severity indices. AMIA Jt Summits Transl Sci Proc 2018; 2017:310–9.

42. Wilkes EH, Rumsby G, Woodward GM. Using machine learning to aid the interpretation of urine steroid profiles. Clin Chem 2018;64(11):1586–95.

43. Wilkes EH, Emmett E, Beltran L, et al. A machine learning approach for the automated interpretation of plasma amino acid profiles. Clin Chem 2020;66(9): 1210–8.

44. Eisenhofer G, Duran C, Cannistraci CV, et al. Use of steroid profiling combined with machine learning for identification and subtype classification in primary aldosteronism. JAMA Netw Open 2020;3(9):e2016209.

45. Laengsri V, Shoombuatong W, Adirojananon W, et al. ThalPred: a web-based prediction tool for discriminating thalassemia trait and iron deficiency anemia. BMC Med Inform Decis Mak 2019;19(1):212.

46. Weis C, Cuenod A, Rieck B, et al. Direct antimicrobial resistance prediction from clinical MALDI-TOF mass spectra using machine learning. Nat Med 2022;28(1): 164–74.

47. Feretzakis G, Sakagianni A, Loupelis E, et al. Machine learning for antibiotic resistance prediction: a prototype using off-the-shelf techniques and entry-level data to guide empiric antimicrobial therapy. Healthc Inform Res 2021;27(3):214–21.

48. Tzelves L, Lazarou L, Feretzakis G, et al. Using machine learning techniques to predict antimicrobial resistance in stone disease patients. World J Urol 2022. https://doi.org/10.1007/s00345-022-04043-x.

49. Waljee AK, Sauder K, Patel A, et al. Machine learning algorithms for objective remission and clinical outcomes with thiopurines. J Crohns Colitis 2017;11(7): 801–10.

50. Hawker CD, McCarthy W, Cleveland D, et al. Invention and validation of an automated camera system that uses optical character recognition to identify patient name mislabeled samples. Clin Chem 2014;60(3):463–70.
51. Oyaert M, Delanghe J. Progress in automated urinalysis. Ann Lab Med 2019; 39(1):15–22.
52. U.S. Food and Drug Administration. DIP/U.S. Urine analysis test system K173327 approval letter. 2018. Available at: https://www.accessdata.fda.gov/cdrh_docs/pdf17/K173327.pdf. Accessed July 5, 2022.
53. Smith GT, Dwork N, Khan SA, et al. Robust dipstick urinalysis using a low-cost, micro-volume slipping manifold and mobile phone platform. Lab Chip 2016; 16(11):2069–78.
54. Bakan E, Bayraktutan Z, Baygutalp NK, et al. Evaluation of the analytical performances of Cobas 6500 and Sysmex UN series automated urinalysis systems with manual microscopic particle counting. Biochem Med (Zagreb) 2018;28(2): 020712.
55. Liang Y, Kang R, Lian C, et al. An end-to-end system for automatic urinary particle recognition with convolutional neural network. J Med Syst 2018;42(9):165.
56. Ince FD, Ellidag HY, Koseoglu M, et al. The comparison of automated urine analyzers with manual microscopic examination for urinalysis automated urine analyzers and manual urinalysis. Pract Lab Med 2016;5:14–20.
57. Laiwejpithaya S, Wongkrajang P, Reesukumal K, et al. UriSed 3 and UX-2000 automated urine sediment analyzers vs manual microscopic method: a comparative performance analysis. J Clin Lab Anal 2018;32(2). https://doi.org/10.1002/jcla.22249.
58. Linko S, Kouri TT, Toivonen E, et al. Analytical performance of the Iris iQ200 automated urine microscopy analyzer. Clin Chim Acta 2006;372(1–2):54–64.
59. Durant TJS, Olson EM, Schulz WL, et al. Very deep convolutional neural networks for morphologic classification of erythrocytes. Clin Chem 2017;63(12):1847–55.
60. Chandradevan R, Aljudi AA, Drumheller BR, et al. Machine-based detection and classification for bone marrow aspirate differential counts: initial development focusing on nonneoplastic cells. Lab Invest 2020;100(1):98–109.
61. Durant TJS, Dudgeon SN, McPadden J, et al. Applications of digital microscopy and densely connected convolutional neural networks for automated quantification of babesia-infected erythrocytes. Clin Chem 2021;68(1):218–29.
62. Satoh M, Vazquez-Del Mercado M, Chan EK. Clinical interpretation of antinuclear antibody tests in systemic rheumatic diseases. Mod Rheumatol 2009;19(3): 219–28.
63. De Bruyne S, Speeckaert MM, Van Biesen W, et al. Recent evolutions of machine learning applications in clinical laboratory medicine. Crit Rev Clin Lab Sci 2021; 58(2):131–52.
64. Park Y, Kim SY, Kwon GC, et al. Automated versus conventional microscopic interpretation of antinuclear antibody indirect immunofluorescence test. Ann Clin Lab Sci 2019;49(1):127–33.
65. Nagy G, Csipo I, Tarr T, et al. Anti-neutrophil cytoplasmic antibody testing by indirect immunofluorescence: computer-aided versus conventional microscopic evaluation of routine diagnostic samples from patients with vasculitis or other inflammatory diseases. Clin Chim Acta 2020;511:117–24.
66. Wu YD, Sheu RK, Chung CW, et al. Application of supervised machine learning to recognize competent level and mixed antinuclear antibody patterns based on ICAP international consensus. Diagnostics (Basel) 2021;11(4). https://doi.org/10.3390/diagnostics11040642.

67. Punchoo R, Bhoora S, Pillay N. Applications of machine learning in the chemical pathology laboratory. J Clin Pathol 2021;74(7):435–42.

68. Li H, Racine-Brzostek S, Xi N, Luo J, Zhao Z, Yuan J. Learning to Detect Monoclonal Protein in Electrophoresis Images. 2021 International Conference on Visual Communications and Image Processing (VCIP). 2021:1-5. doi:10.1109/VCIP53242.2021.9675332

69. Wei XY, Yang ZQ, Zhang XL, et al. Deep collocative learning for immunofixation electrophoresis image analysis. IEEE Trans Med Imaging 2021;40(7):1898–910.

70. Chabrun F, Dieu X, Ferre M, et al. Achieving expert-level interpretation of serum protein electrophoresis through deep learning driven by human reasoning. Clin Chem 2021;67(10):1406–14.

71. Santilli AML, Ren K, Oleschuk R, et al. Application of intraoperative mass spectrometry and data analytics for oncological margin detection, a review. IEEE Trans Biomed Eng 2022;69(7):2220–32.

72. Kim JI, Maguire F, Tsang KK, et al. Machine learning for antimicrobial resistance prediction: current practice, limitations, and clinical perspective. Clin Microbiol Rev 2022;e0017921. https://doi.org/10.1128/cmr.00179-21.

73. Vicente FB, Lin DC, Haymond S. Automation of chromatographic peak review and order to result data transfer in a clinical mass spectrometry laboratory. Clin Chim Acta 2019;498:84–9.

74. Eilertz D, Mitterer M, Buescher JM. automRm: an r package for fully automatic LC-QQQ-MS data preprocessing powered by machine learning. Anal Chem 2022;94(16):6163–71.

75. Yu M, Bazydlo LAL, Bruns DE, et al. Streamlining quality review of mass spectrometry data in the clinical laboratory by use of machine learning. Arch Pathol Lab Med 2019;143(8):990–8.

76. Peng G, Tang Y, Cowan TM, et al. Reducing false-positive results in newborn screening using machine learning. Int J Neonatal Screen 2020;6(1). https://doi.org/10.3390/ijns6010016.

77. Subhashini P, Jaya Krishna S, Usha Rani G, et al. Application of machine learning algorithms for the differential diagnosis of peroxisomal disorders. J Biochem 2019;165(1):67–73.

78. Labriffe M, Woillard JB, Debord J, et al. Machine learning algorithms to estimate everolimus exposure trained on simulated and patient pharmacokinetic profiles. CPT Pharmacometrics Syst Pharmacol 2022. https://doi.org/10.1002/psp4.12810.

79. Woillard JB, Labriffe M, Debord J, et al. Mycophenolic acid exposure prediction using machine learning. Clin Pharmacol Ther 2021;110(2):370–9.

80. Burghelea D, Moisoiu T, Ivan C, et al. The use of machine learning algorithms and the mass spectrometry lipidomic profile of serum for the evaluation of tacrolimus exposure and toxicity in kidney transplant recipients. Biomedicines 2022;10(5). https://doi.org/10.3390/biomedicines10051157.

81. Chary M, Boyer EW, Burns MM. Diagnosis of Acute Poisoning using explainable artificial intelligence. Comput Biol Med 2021;134:104469.

82. Randell EW, Yenice S, Khine Wamono AA, et al. Autoverification of test results in the core clinical laboratory. Clin Biochem 2019;73:11–25.

83. Demirci F, Akan P, Kume T, et al. Artificial neural network approach in laboratory test reporting: learning algorithms. Am J Clin Pathol 2016;146(2):227–37. https://doi.org/10.1093/ajcp/aqw104.

84. Wang H, Wang H, Zhang J, et al. Using machine learning to develop an autover-ification system in a clinical biochemistry laboratory. Clin Chem Lab Med 2021; 59(5):883–91.
85. Hoffmann RG. Statistics in the practice of medicine. JAMA 1963;185:864–73.
86. Bhattacharya CG. A simple method of resolution of a distribution into Gaussian components. Biometrics 1967;23(1):115–35.
87. Jones GRD, Haeckel R, Loh TP, et al. Indirect methods for reference interval determination - review and recommendations. Clin Chem Lab Med 2018; 57(1):20–9.
88. Poole S, Schroeder LF, Shah N. An unsupervised learning method to identify reference intervals from a clinical database. J Biomed Inform 2016;59:276–84.
89. Yang Q, Mwenda KM, Ge M. Incorporating geographical factors with artificial neural networks to predict reference values of erythrocyte sedimentation rate. Int J Health Geogr 2013;12:11.
90. Jackson BR, Ye Y, Crawford JM, et al. The ethics of artificial intelligence in pathology and laboratory medicine: principles and practice. Acad Pathol 2021;8. https://doi.org/10.1177/2374289521990784. 2374289521990784.
91. Schulz WL, Durant TJS, Krumholz HM. Validation and regulation of clinical artificial intelligence. Clin Chem 2019;65(10):1336–7.
92. Char DS, Abramoff MD, Feudtner C. Identifying ethical considerations for machine learning healthcare applications. Am J Bioeth 2020;20(11):7–17.
93. Vayena E, Blasimme A, Cohen IG. Machine learning in medicine: addressing ethical challenges. PLoS Med 2018;15(11):e1002689.
94. Mahajan SM, Heidenreich P, Abbott B, et al. Predictive models for identifying risk of readmission after index hospitalization for heart failure: a systematic review. Eur J Cardiovasc Nurs 2018;17(8):675–89.
95. Marin MJ, Van Wijk XMR, Durant TJS. Machine learning in healthcare: mapping a path to title 21. Clin Chem 2022;68(4):609–10.
96. Wilson FP, Martin M, Yamamoto Y, et al. Electronic health record alerts for acute kidney injury: multicenter, randomized clinical trial. BMJ 2021;372:m4786.
97. Lachance P, Villeneuve PM, Rewa OG, et al. Association between e-alert implementation for detection of acute kidney injury and outcomes: a systematic review. Nephrol Dial Transpl 2017;32(2):265–72.
98. Obermeyer Z, Powers B, Vogeli C, et al. Dissecting racial bias in an algorithm used to manage the health of populations. Science 2019;366(6464):447–53.

Digital Health
Today's Solutions and Tomorrow's Impact

Alison Hellmann, BS[a],*, Ashley Emmons, MS[a],
Matthew Stewart Prime, BSc, MBBS, PhD, MRCS(Eng)[b],
Ketan Paranjape, PhD, MBA[a], Denise L. Heaney, PhD[a]

KEYWORDS

- Artificial intelligence • Clinical decision support • Clinical algorithms
- Digital health solutions • Digital diagnostics • Digital health care innovation

KEY POINTS

- Artificial intelligence (AI) is becoming an indispensable tool to augment decision making in different healthcare settings.
- The role of the patient is evolving and digital health solutions and AI can help to empower the patient to take an active role in their healthcare decisions.
- AI cannot replace the clinician in patient care, however, those who do not adopt AI may in time, be left behind.
- There are many examples of digital health solutions that leverage AI today to enable more informed clinical decisions.
- AI in healthcare is still evolving and will play an even more critical role in future.

INTRODUCTION TO ARTIFICIAL INTELLIGENCE FOR DIGITAL HEALTH SOLUTIONS

As the digital health care transformation unfolds, artificial intelligence (AI), algorithms, and clinical decision support are becoming a more accepted and integrated part of the health care ecosystem. Laboratory results and the decisions that are based on them are taking place outside the walls of the laboratory, clinic, and hospital. Digital health care came to life globally through the COVID-19 pandemic, and a compound annual growth of 15.1% is projected each year from 2021 to 2028.[1] Another significant shift is in the role of patients in their own health care journeys and decisions.

In this article, we are going to focus on emerging digital health solutions that include those that use AI to provide clinical decision support. Using specific examples, we will cover how these technologies are changing how and where health care decisions are made today and how they will continue to disrupt health care in the future.

[a] Roche Diagnostics, 9115 Hague Road, Indianapolis, IN 46256, USA; [b] Roche Information Solutions, Kornfeldstrasse 42, Riehen 4125, Basel Stadt, Switzerland
* Corresponding author.
E-mail address: ali.hellmann@roche.com

Clin Lab Med 43 (2023) 71–86
https://doi.org/10.1016/j.cll.2022.09.006
labmed.theclinics.com

Digital health is a broad term with a vast scope. It can include categories such as mobile health, health information technology, wearable devices, telehealth, telemedicine, and personalized medicine. Digital health solutions are regulated based on the potential risk they pose to patients.

Traditionally in a health care system, when thinking about digital solutions, Health IT systems like Electronic Health Records (EHR) or Electronic Medical Record (EMR), Laboratory Information Systems (LIS), Hospital Information Systems (HIS), and middleware tend to come to mind. Although these systems are the digital backbone of information in US health care systems, they are not the focus of this article. Instead, we will focus on AI and how it can optimize data to provide clinical decision support for clinicians and laboratorians and/or empower patients to play an active role in their own health care journey.

VALUE OF AI IN LABORATORY MEDICINE

AI is becoming an indispensable tool to augment decision making in various health care settings. For example, AI is commonly used in the clinical laboratory to automate microscopic CBC differentials and urine sediment examinations to substantially reduce the need for manual technologist review. Likewise, AI-based algorithms have been trained to diagnose a wide variety of clinical disorders such as multimyeloma and iron deficiency anemia. See **Table 1** for additional examples.

As laboratory medicine evolves post the COVID-19 pandemic, given the surge in the volume of tests being run in a constrained environment of staff shortages, there is a need for the laboratories to undergo automation and digitization by introducing technologies like AI.

We recently conducted a survey to explore the current perceptions, usage, and anticipated challenges related to the use of AI in diagnostics laboratories. We compared results from our recent survey to a similar survey [1] from 2019 with the intent of understanding how much progress has been made and how sentiment/value proposition has changed in the last 3 years. The current survey collected quantitative responses to 26 questions from 139 participants followed by an asynchronous discussion forum with 112 participants. See **Table 1** for sample details.

Key observations from this recent survey included:

1. AI's perceived value to health care and diagnostics has increased significantly and across multiple areas between 2019 and 2022
   a. Although the usage of AI in diagnostics has not significantly increased between 2019 and 2022, the perceived value of AI in both general health care applications and diagnostics has increased
      i. When posed with a list of challenges in health care and asked for their opinion on the value of AI in these areas, all T2B categories are up compared to 2019, with most notable increases in perceived value for laboratory consolidations (58% in 2022) and fee-for-value contracts (68% in 2022)
      ii. The perceived value of AI specifically in diagnostics has increased significantly from 2019 to 2022 (+22%), with 67% of participants believing AI will be either extremely valuable or very valuable
         1. Molecular, hematology & hemostasis, and urinalysis were specific diagnostic areas that saw statistically significant increases.
   b. Participants would like to see AI play a role in increasing laboratory efficiencies, data processing, and administrative support
   c. A minority of participants are skeptical regarding the value of AI; some have difficulty seeing how AI would address these challenges, while others are hesitant toward new technology

d. The current environment created by COVID-19 encourages swift adoption of new, efficiency-driving technologies for 49% of participants organizations, and creates resource-driven barriers for 28% of participants organizations

2. For AI to be successfully implemented in any given organization, engaging the right stakeholders, and increasing AI-specific training/education is critical
   a. Participants see Administrators/Leadership, IT, and Finance as the most critical stakeholders to involve for AI-related decisions
      i. Participants see increased importance in the role of IT and Finance for AI implementation, with 75% of Advisors noting the importance of IT (up from 63% in 2019), and 60% noting the importance of Finance, up from 47% in 2019
   b. When it comes to training and education around AI, participants expect support from manufacturer and platform providers, inclusion of AI-related topics in medical professional education, and even potentially AI-specific teams and roles

Table 1

Table 1 Selected illustrative examples involving applications of AI to health care; survey sample information (n = 139)		
Test Performed	**AI Technique Applied**	**Outcomes**
Discriminate between positive and negative urine tests[2]	Supervised ML, Classification and Regression Tree (CART)	Better classifiers can reduce microscopic review rates by 30% and decrease significant losses in urinalysis
Predicting human age[3]	Deep neural networks	Found albumin concentration followed by glucose best identified age. Identified 5 markers (albumin, glucose, alkaline phosphate, urea, and erythrocytes) as the most valuable to predicting human age
Predicting Type 2 diabetes[4]	Supervised ML, L1-regularized, logistical regression	Combined administrative claims, pharmacy records, health care utilization, laboratory results. Identified surrogate risk factors such as chronic liver disease (odds ratio [OR] 3.71), High alanine aminotransferase (OR 2.26), esophageal reflux (OR 1.85), history of acute bronchitis (OR 1.45).
Predictor for traumatic brain injury[5]	Logistic Regression, Relevance Vector Machine (RVM)	Predicted TBI outcome from laboratory data. Found creatinine level was a clear predictor of outcome of traumatic brain injury. Glucose, albumin, and osmolarity levels were also good predictors

(continued on next page)

Table 1 (*continued*)		
Test Performed	**AI Technique Applied**	**Outcomes**
Discover rheumatoid arthritis[6]	Linear kernel support vector machine, NLP	Combined clinical narratives and laboratory values from electronic medical records (EMRs) to identify responders and nonresponders for pharmacogenomics research
Warfarin adequacy, drug-drug interactions[7]	C4.5 decision tree, Random forest	Laboratory tests, alanine aminotransferase (ALT) and serum creatinine (SCr) combined with EHR data – warfarin dose, gender, age, and weight. Automated results were "more accurate than clinical physicians' subjective decision"
Hematological disease diagnosis[8]	Support vector machine (SVM), Naïve Bayesian Classifier, Random forest	Applying ML on laboratory blood test results can predict hematologic disease – prediction accuracies of 0.88 and 0.86 for 5 most likely diseases (multiple myeloma, amyloidosis, iron deficiency anemia, Purpura)

INDUSTRY DEVELOPED VERSUS HOMEGROWN BY A HEALTH CARE SYSTEM

When health care institutions decide to pursue digital tools for decision making, an important consideration is whether they build the tools themselves (homegrown) or buy it.

Key reasons to build internally include options to address all your requirements the best way possible, full control and flexibility including control on costs. What institutions lack is internal expertise and ability to quantify the effort needed to build solutions that can scale with increase in demand, and the inability to run the development effort like a software company.

Buying custom off-the-shelf software covers most of your requirements, reduces your total cost of ownership, and gives you an ability to quantify the expense as operational with the added benefit that the vendor manages all the enhancements and upgrades. On the cons side, you have less flexibility and control, depend on the delivery schedule of the vendor, and are locked into cost and interoperability.

In a nutshell, the key drivers are control and cost. Then, when it comes to making a decision, the question to answer is ownership—do you have true ownership of the solution and is the total cost of ownership economically sustainable?

SPEED OF DEVELOPMENT

Technology has changed the world over in the past decades and we are starting to see the digital transformation in health care take shape. In 1950, it was estimated that medical knowledge doubled in 50 years. In 1980 that time shortened to 7 years, and in 2011, it was estimated that by 2020 medical knowledge would double in just 73 days.[9] In 2018, John Rumsfeld, MD, PhD, FACC, ACC's Chief Innovation Officer, stated, "We're right at the beginning of what is likely to be a revolution in healthcare delivery, but we're struggling in the adoption of digital technologies."[10] The COVID-19 pandemic expedited the development of health care innovation. What previously would take years to develop and bring to market progressed at an unprecedented rate.

An an example of this speed of innovation over the past 2 years, consider the COVID-19 Map, created by Lauren Gardner and her team at Johns Hopkins University, that launched in January of 2020.[11] This dashboard became the single source of truth regarding the state of the pandemic. It was used to inform about the rapidly spreading virus so critical decisions could be made, and it brought to light insights regarding health care disparities. This important tool was developed in only a matter of months by a team of people collecting, verifying, and communicating data in a way that is easy to understand. **Fig. 1**

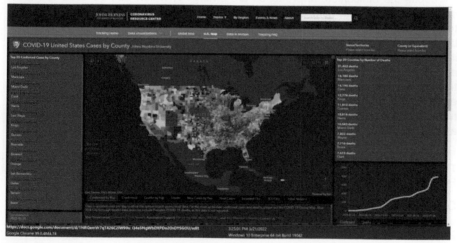

Fig. 1. Screenshot of the COVID-19 United States cases by County Map by Johns Hopkins University, as captured on 21 March 2022.[11]

Another instance of innovation we saw emerge from the COVID-19 pandemic relates to the trend of virtual care, telehealth, and remote patient monitoring. Until recently, these technologies were frequent topics of discussion and scholarly publication but had relatively scant real-world adoption. The start of the pandemic ushered a rapid transformation from hospital-based services and physician offices to in-home care and retail clinics. Digital health was a rapidly advancing trend early in the pandemic. The advancement, promotion, and subsequent adoption of telemedicine that materialized from the onslaught of COVID-19 is a prime example. Innovation for digital health care solutions is quickly being developed, tested, and frequently even accepted for COVID-19 and beyond.

EVIDENCE GENERATION FOR DIGITAL HEALTH SOLUTIONS

Despite the ability for digital health solutions to be developed and tested rapidly, full and widespread adoption remains a challenge. For successful innovation diffusion, a solution must demonstrate a relative advantage as compared to existing options.[12] In the context of digital health solutions (incl. AI solutions), this can be (1) clinical benefit (eg, improved clinical outcome), (2) operational efficiency (eg, reduced administrative tasks), (3) financial value (eg, prevention of readmission penalties), and (4) user-experience (eg, improved patient and clinician satisfaction). Ideally, a solution should offer value in all dimensions, but importantly it should not improve value in one dimension at the expense of another.

When we consider digital health solutions (incl. AI solutions), there are 3 critical evidence stakeholders: the regulator—focus on safety & quality of solution; the end-user—focus on clinical utility & user-experience; and the buyer—focus on operational & financial impacts.

Each stakeholder has a different focus and, as such, innovators must generate multiple types of evidence. In health care, the traditional and expected method to evaluate an intervention is by clinical trial, which normally evaluates an unchanging intervention, such as a drug. Such approaches are ill-suited for digital health solutions due to the rapid development process and continuous version updates.[13] This challenge can be even greater for AI-based solutions, such as learning algorithms, which can change based on new inputs.

Despite the difficulties, approaches are emerging, which can be used to rapidly evaluate digital health solutions. Computational simulation is regularly used to test the generalizability of AI solutions for different contexts, and clinical simulation has been used to test the user experience, operational impacts, and clinical utility for digital health workflow solutions. Notwithstanding, these techniques require robust aggregate and/or individual-level clinical data to test the solutions sufficiently. In addition, future efforts should incorporate continuous real-world data evaluations to ensure impacts are sustained overtime, and to highlight where solutions can be optimized further. Equally important is that evidence stakeholders (ie, regulators, users, and buyers) are open-minded to what and how evidence is generated.

TYPES OF DIGITAL HEALTH SOLUTIONS: PROVIDER-FOCUSED VERSUS PATIENT-FOCUSED

One may choose to categorize digital health solutions as provider-focused (intended for use by health care providers) or patient-focused (intended for direct use by patients). Patient-focused solutions may include hardware and software, including smartphone apps, designed to monitor or collect patient data and/or to support patient health care decision making. For example, digital health solutions may include apps such as sleep and activity trackers, cardiac monitors, digital interfaces for home laboratory tests, and applications designed to help patients communicate with their clinicians and make decisions about their health. In many cases, patient-focused solutions would benefit from EHR integration, both to enable them to obtain accurate and detailed patient health information and to allow them to communicate monitoring and other data back to health care providers. Patient-focused solutions can sometimes include AI-based algorithms that can detect trends and changes in trends. In certain circumstances, having awareness of significant changes in trends may prompt a patient to contact their health care provider for guidance. In addition, many of these tools have education included, providing the patient the ability to interact as well as learn about their disease state, thus empowering the patient to make decisions that can have an impact on their own positive outcomes. In the following sections, we will explore various and diverse examples, one of which will be a digital solution called iThemba Life, which includes a dashboard for health care providers to examine trends in the data of their patient population and find insights for providers and program managers.

Some digital solutions are made specifically for health care providers. These tools may pull data from various sources that are already live in the health care system, for instance from the LIS, EHR, and NAVIFY imaging files, then display the information in a single platform designed for easier interpretation. One of the following examples, NAVIFY Tumor Board (NTB), is a space that was built for the purposes of collaboration between HCPs.

Patient-Focused Examples

Patient engagement and empowerment while expanding access to quality care: iThemba Life

The 95-95-95 Joint United Nations Program on HIV/AIDS is an initiative to end the AIDS epidemic by the year 2030 by achieving viral suppression for 95% of people living with HIV. As of 2018, 19% of South Africans were living with HIV, and despite having treatments for HIV, only 86% of people living with HIV successfully achieved viral suppression. Although viral load (VL) testing is increasing, there is a challenge with adherence to medications and the continuum of care. When explored, a problem was identified related to the delivery of health care and information. VL test results are delayed, which then causes a delay in clinical decision making leading to the challenge in achieving program results.

To help solve these challenges, Roche sought to develop a cloud-based tool that would promote patient engagement during HIV care and can be integrated with local laboratory information systems or results databases. Roche developed and piloted this tool in South Africa, which hosts the largest HIV Treatment Program in the world. Starting with a concept and prototype, Roche sought feedback by partnering with more than 40 health care professionals and more than 60 people living with HIV (PLWH) in South Africa. Roche iterated the product based on feedback and developed iThemba Life. iThemba Life is not available in the United States.

iThemba user interfaces were developed to ensure results were displayed in a way that was easy for the participant to understand and that if actions were required, they were clear. This included use of a traffic-light display to contextualize results: A green results screen means the results are good and keep taking your medication, yellow means the virus is not suppressed and a reminder to take medication properly is displayed, and red indicates the need to visit the clinic immediately because the virus is present and growing fast. **Fig. 2**

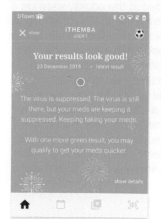
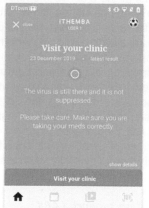
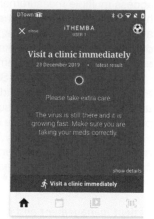

Fig. 2. Screenshot of in-app laboratory results explanations. (https://formative.jmir.org/2022/2/e26033 JMIR Form Res 2022 | vol. 6 | iss. 2 |e26033 |p. 3.)

Roche conducted a study in Johannesburg, South Africa, to assess the impact of iThemba Life in the time to HIV VL results delivery compared to the time of results delivery before iThemba Life. Roche also tested the feasibility and acceptability from patients of using iThemba Life to receive their HIV VL results.

The conclusion of the study showed that iThemba Life was well-received by participants, despite limited smartphone access for some.[14] Regarding time to results delivery, iThemba Life app users received their results 10 times faster compared to delivery before use with iThemba Life (6 days vs 56 days) and 5 times faster compared to before use with iThemba Life if the results showed their virus was not suppressed (7 days vs 37.5 days).[14] The faster turnaround time of results delivery notification translated to participants wanting to continue use of iThemba Life.

It is important to note that iThemba Life was developed through a collaboration between industry and frontline health care providers. Through this partnership, a challenge was identified, workflows and information flows were assessed, the patient and provider experiences were explored. This approach allowed for the development of a solution, iThemba Life, that has the potential to assist with compliance to care and patient understanding. Future studies are needed to assess the impact of iThemba Life on patient outcomes.[14]

Wearables for continuous, remote monitoring

Wearables are a source of personal health care data, and the market was valued at $16.6 billion in 2020. The market is expected to grow with a compound annual growth rate of 26.8% from 2021 to 2028.[15] Siren is a company that developed a wearable digital solution in a sock.

Diabetic foot ulcers (DFU) occur in approximately 25% of diabetics. Many times, severe DFU can lead to complications and amputation. Early detection and intervention of DFU can notably reduce the risk of pain and reduce the risk of amputation in severe cases.[16] Diabetic neuropathy contributes to the risk of DFU development. Measuring skin temperature in the foot has been shown to reduce the risk of DFU. However, traditional tools measure skin temperature of the foot at points in time, such as when visiting the doctor.

Siren is a company that developed a smart sock for patients with diabetes. The socks are designed to be used daily, and they continuously monitor the skin temperature foot of the person with diabetes through sensors that are embedded throughout.[16]

In 2018, Siren conducted a study to show that the sensors in the socks were able to access multiple measurements of the 6 sensors embedded in the socks, showing a high level of agreement to the reference standard. Patients assessed the comfort level and ease of use of the socks, finding a median score of 9 or 10 on a 10-point scale. The data showed the smart socks are able to compare the temperature of the wearer's feet and inform the wearer of temperature increases through the use of a mobile app.[16]

Since the study in 2018, Siren developed a hub that patients plug in at home. This hub allows health care providers to have access to the data generated from the continuously monitoring smart socks without the need for a patient to use a smartphone.[17–19] Siren socks are sometimes covered by insurance and medicare.[17–19]

Incorporating technology, like that of Siren's smart socks, to continuously and remotely monitor the temperature of a diabetic patient's feet has the potential to facilitate early detection and timely intervention of foot ulcers, thereby reducing the risk of complications from DFUs.[16]

Patient management and decision support: LARK

Type 2 diabetes is a health condition that affects more than 37 million people in the United States.[20] Often, this chronic health condition can be managed by the patient through lifestyle changes including healthy eating habits, being active, and blood sugar management.[20] Although lifestyle changes are important for managing diabetes, patients often struggle to manage this condition without guidance from a physician. Economic resources for managing type 2 diabetes are also sparse regarding behavioral changes and weight management.[21] With technology, such as AI, patient-centered care that is economically sustainable is possible. Michigan State University performed a longitudinal observational study including 70 participants who had a body mass index $\geq$ 25 kg/m^2 using the Lark Weight Loss Health Coach AI (HCAI). The study evaluated the participants' weight loss, changes in meal quality, and app acceptability among participants.[21] Over the course of 15 weeks, participants in this study averaged a 2.4 kg weight loss.[21] There was an improvement in dietary pattern, the participants' healthy meals logged increased by 31% and unhealthy meals decreased by 54%.[21] The study also showed that using a mobile phone application to deliver conversational AI had high acceptability among participants. The application had a satisfaction score of 87% and a net promoter score of 47.[21] The results of this study showed that the use of AI can result in weight loss and increased healthy lifestyle behaviors that are associated with reduced diabetes risk.[21]

Using remote patient monitoring to expand access to care: locus health

The National Pediatric Cardiology Quality Improvement Collaboration (NPC-QIC) formed in 2006 with the mission "to decrease mortality and improving quality of life for infants with single ventricle congenital heart disease and their families."[23] The NPC-QIC developed an interstate home monitoring program to help increase the chances of survival for these very at-risk babies between surgeries 1 and 2 of the 3 phase palliation procedure. The program, initially aimed at early identification of risk, such as decreased oxygen saturation and acute weight loss or failure to gain weight after stage 1, has evolved with technology over time.[22,23] Today, NPC-QIC patients have a 95% chance of surviving the interstage period.[22] **Fig. 3**

To explore how, let's look at what happened in 2017 when Riley Children's Hospital in Indianapolis, a member of NPC-QIC since 2009, incorporated Locus software into their remote monitoring solution.[24] Locus is a software platform that allows for real-time collaboration of patients/parents and the care team as well as remote monitoring of important health information when a patient is discharged from the hospital. Riley and Locus collaborated to develop a solution for parents of patients that can be used between the first and second stages of surgery. The collaboration resulted in parents bringing home their babies with specific direction and means to monitor and communicate with the care team at Riley. Parents were sent home with tools to monitor SPO2, weight, heart rate, emesis, intake and output, and medication tracking.[24] Today, parents are also sent home with an iPad that includes the Locus app. These tools allow parents of these high-risk cardiac babies to, as one parent put it, "Have the Riley team in my back pocket."[25]

Incorporating the solution impacted the amount of patients Riley can care for in a positive way. In 1 year, Riley went from monitoring 10 patients remotely to monitoring 31, without the need to hire additional staff, through the use of the Locus platform. In 2019, Riley expanded their monitoring program to other high-risk patients as well. Patients are able to provide feedback via surveys in the Locus app. Through these surveys, parents rate the solution strongly on feeling:

- Confident they can provide care at home to their child
- Comfortable leaving the hospital with their child
- Connected to my care team[24]

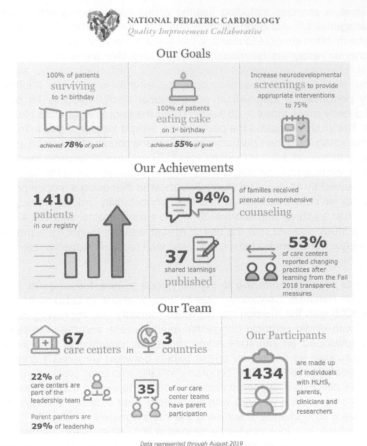

Fig. 3. Infographic explaining the success of NPC-QIC.23

This partnership is a great example of health care data being generated to impact decisions for patients, all outside hospital and laboratory walls. It also shows that with the right tools, patients, or in this case parents, can be confident, empowered, and connected to take an active role in the health care plan.

Provider-Focused Examples

The use of algorithms to help find what the eye may not see

Measuring pain is not an easy task because of its varied and subjective nature.[26] In a study focused on osteoarthritis of the knee, pain levels were found to be higher in underserved populations, even after controlling for objective severity, as graded by human physicians assessing pain using medical images. It was hypothesized that this disparity was due to external factors, such as stress. However, an algorithm was developed that uses knee x-rays to predict a patients' experienced pain. When comparing this algorithmic approach to standard measures of severity graded by radiologists, the algorithm showed reductions in unexplained racial disparities in pain (43% vs 9%). The data suggest that much of the pain reported in underserved populations is generated from factors within the knee that are not reflected in standard x-ray imaging, rather than from disparities rooted in racial and socioeconomic diversity. The information gathered from this study is an example of how taking an algorithmic approach to assess knee pain has the potential to influence measurement, assessment, and treatment decisions for patients.[27]**Fig. 4**

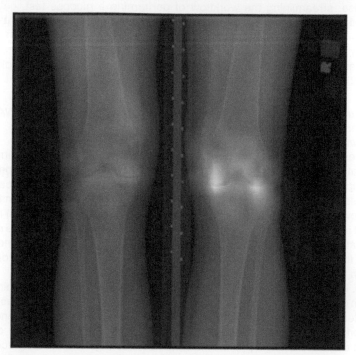

Fig. 4. Heatmap of a representative x-ray image. The model's prediction target is the pain score in the knee appearing on the right side of the image. Regions that influence the predictions are more strongly shown in brighter colors.[27]

Bringing clinical decision support to the point of care

One-third of all hospitalized patients require insulin therapy during their stay. In November of 2021, CMS introduced 3 new electronic quality measures, 2 of them related to inpatient glycemic management:

- Requirement: report rates of severe hyperglycemia during a hospital stay
- Mandate: data on patients experiencing severe hypoglycemia, which is intended to identify preventable medication-induced hypoglycemia[28]

Glytec is the provider of Glucommander, a clinical decision support software for inpatient glycemic management. Glucommander has been shown to reduce low blood sugar by 99.8%, 30-day readmissions by 36% to 68%, and length of stay by up to 3.2 days.[29]

cobas pulse, a product that is not available in the United States, was developed to be an automated data collection and information management system through the ability to run third-party applications on the device. cobas pulse system will also be the next generation Point of Care (POC) glucose testing system by Roche. In a sense, the device is designed to be a hospital-grade smart device with high levels of security that also performs glucose testing at the bedside. Combining a glucose meter with a smart device, cobas pulse may enable care teams to streamline workflows by having access to information and clinical decision support software at the Point of Care.

In January of 2022, Roche announced a partnership with Gytec. This partnership would allow for Glytec's Glucommander software to be available as an app on cobas pulse, streamlining the workflow of performing a glucose test, getting the result, and deciding what to do next to effectively manage the patient's blood glucose. Bringing the clinical decision support of Glucommander onto cobas pulse, a device that could oftentimes be in within reach of the nurse and care team, can help address the challenges related to inpatient glucose management directly at the patient's bedside.[28]

Digital solutions centralizing desperate data and fostering collaboration: NAVIFY Tumor Board & NAVIFY Oncology Hub
NAVIFY Tumor Board.

Cancer is one of the leading causes of death worldwide, resulting in approximately 10 million deaths in 2020.[30] A tumor board is a meeting that is composed of physicians from multiple disciplines coming together to review a patient's full medical history and discussing the best treatment options for that patient's cancer based on their collective knowledge and experience.[31] Multidisciplinary tumor boards (MTBs) require a significant amount of time and preparation from each specialty for each case review.[32] Approximately 47% of health care systems report that their oncologists spend 2 hours preparing for a complex case review, whereas other specialists report spending up to 6 hours on case preparation.[32]

In 2016, Roche collaborated with the Hospital del Mar in Barcelona, Spain, for the cocreation of a digital tumor board solution, NTB, to address the obstacles associated with the tumor board preparation process. NTB is an efficiency-enhancing cloud-based workflow product that supports MTB meetings. Through NTB, an oncology care team can have a single platform to schedule meetings and securely access, review, and share patient data. MTB members are able to review patient data and current therapies before the meeting using Clinical Decision Support (CDS) applications that are integrated into the NTB software.[32]

An observational study was conducted that included[33]:

- 2 surgeons
- 2 oncologists
- 2 pathologists
- 2 radiologists

The study compared preparation of current tumor board practices to preparation using NTB for breast cancer cases. At the conclusion of the study, a significant reduction in case preparation was seen among surgeons, oncologists, and radiologists. There was a significant decrease in clinical course data review and other preparation tasks, but pathology and radiology review did not differ significantly. A survey among users in the study indicated that NTB had higher ratings than the current tumor board method on all ease of use and satisfaction survey questions. This study supported the hypothesis that a digital solution improves tumor board case preparation. Future studies in different cancer types, hospitals, and with more physicians would be required to assess the impact of NTB.

In addition, in collaboration with the University of Missouri, the impact of NTB on tumor board preparation time was evaluated across multiple user groups in 4 cancer categories; hematopathology, breast, head and neck, and GI cancer. The study was designed to compare tumor board preparation for multiple hospital staff during 4 phases; pre-NTB, after implementation of manual NTB (no integration with hospital EMR), initial/partial integration with EMR followed by pathology report integration, and the stable phase after the completion of integration.[34]

The results of this study indicate that NTB has a significant impact on case preparation. The study showed a significant reduction in overall case preparation time (30%).[34] Comparing phase 1 (pre-NTB) to phase 4 (post-NTB) case throughput showed an 82% case per week increase for breast cancer and a 38% increase for GI cancer.[34] There was a 23.5% decrease in hematopathology cancer cases and no significant changes seen in ENT cancer case throughput.[34] 18.3 minutes were saved per breast cancer case, 9.9 minutes per GI cancer case, and 17.4 minutes per ENT cancer case.[34]

NTB standardizes case presentation and discussion during tumor boards and reduces the postponement of case discussion.[34] The study concluded that the impact of NTB on time for case preparation was significant and the improvements were continuous and sustained over time.[34]

NAVIFY Oncology Hub

The adoption of electronic medical records (EMRs) has been linked to physician burnout because of the extensive documentation that is required of clinicians.[35] For every patient contact hour, clinicians report spending an average of 2 hours on the EMR followed by 1 to 2 hours on EMR work at home.[35] EMRs are widely used in the United States and are especially common for oncology care.[36] A cancer patient's journey is complex and can span from months to years; the problem with using EMRs in oncology care is that often the patient data becomes fragmented in the system, making it difficult for a clinician to merge all of this information to make the best treatment decision for the patient.[36] This increased cognitive strain has also been linked to physician burnout.[36]

EMRs also contain nonclinical information, such as billing information. It can be challenging to sift through the various sources of patient health information and to put it together to easily understand all that is happening with a patient. NAVIFY Oncology Hub is a clinical workflow and decision support software that pulls patient information from these disparate sources and brings it together to one platform, creating a holistic view of the patient's clinical journey, enabling easier decision making. This software can allow clinicians to spend less time on paperwork and more time with patients, potentially helping to reduce the challenges leading to physician burnout.

THE FUTURE

We are in the early stages of the digital health revolution, and the role of AI in health care is still taking shape. This revolution has the potential to change the health care experience to have more insightful technology-based and data-driven interactions. The pandemic shined a light on a new demand in the market, and this demand comes from patients, payors, and providers as well. For years, through education and awareness, HCPs have been educating patients more about their own conditions. Now, patients want to also be part of the decision and acquire the tools to be effective. Patients want to be included in the health care ecosystem and advocate for their own wellness. This article discussed examples of digital health solutions that use AI to assist patients in understanding their own health, take ownership of it, and prompt proactive, and potentially life-saving conversations with their care providers.

The examples in this article are inspiring and give hope to how technology and AI can augment decision making in health care. Innovation is happening today. There are challenges we will face related to awareness, adoption, and routine use of these digital health solutions. These challenges should be faced at a place where industry, health care providers, and patients come together to build and define what success looks like. No party can do it alone, as all perspectives are important and should be taken into account. By working together, we have a great opportunity to deliver a health care experience where all parties are informed and empowered to take an active role, an experience that may ultimately enable increased access, reduced costs, and finding ways to improve patient outcomes.

SUMMARY

AI is becoming an indispensable tool to augment decision making in different health care settings and by various members of the patient pathway, including the patient. The pandemic showed us that patients and caregivers want to be empowered to make decisions to impact their own positive outcomes. AI provides the ability to optimize data to bring clinical decision support for clinicians and laboratorians and/or empower patients to actively participate in their own health care. This article discussed many examples of AI and digital health solutions, from those that provide guidance to clinicians to those where the patient is the primary user. Though there are many examples of AI and digital health solutions, the exact role of AI in health care is still being defined. It is becoming clear that although AI cannot replace the clinician, those who do not adopt AI may, in time, be left behind.

DISCLOSURE

This publication was authored by employees of Roche Diagnostics Corporation acting in the scope of their employment. The authors are not subject to any conflicting commercial or financial interests nor are there additional funding sources for this article.

CLINICS CARE POINTS

Artificial intelligence (AI) is becoming an indispensable tool to augment decision making in different health care settings

- The role of the patient is evolving and digital health solutions and AI can help to empower the patient to take an active role in their health care decisions
- AI cannot replace the clinician in patient care; however, those who do not adopt AI may in time, be left behind.
- There are many examples of digital health solutions that leverage AI today to enable more informed clinical decisions.
- AI in health care is still evolving and will play an even more critical role in the future.

REFERENCES

1. Paranjape K, Schinkel M, Hammer RD, et al. The value of artificial intelligence in laboratory medicine. Am J Clin Pathol 2021;155(6):823–31.
2. Yuan C, Ming C, Chengjin H. UrineCART, a machine learning method for establishment of review rules based on UF-1000i flow cytometry and dipstick or reflectance photometer. Clin Chem Lab Med (Cclm) 2012;50(12):2155–61.

3. Putin E, Mamoshina P, Aliper A, et al. Deep biomarkers of human aging: application of deep neural networks to biomarker development. Aging 2016;8(5):1021–33.

4. Razavian N, Blecker S, Schmidt AM, et al. Population-level prediction of type 2 diabetes from Claims data and Analysis of risk factors. Big Data 2015;3(4):277–87.

5. Nelson DW, Rudehill A, MacCallum RM, et al. Multivariate outcome prediction in Traumatic Brain Injury with focus on laboratory values. J Neurotrauma 2012;29(17):2613–24.

6. Lin C, Karlson EW, Canhao H, et al. Automatic prediction of Rheumatoid Arthritis disease activity from the electronic medical records. PLoS ONE 2013;8(8):e69932.

7. Liu KE, Lo CL, Hu YH. Improvement of Adequate Use of Warfarin for the Elderly using decision Tree-based approaches. Methods Inf Med 2014;53(01):47–53.

8. Gunčar G, Kukar M, Notar M, et al. An application of machine learning to haematological diagnosis. Scientific Rep 2018;8(1):411.

9. Densen P. Challenges and opportunities facing medical education. Trans Am Clin Climatol Assoc 2011;122:48–58.

10. Cover story: digital health solutions in cardiovascular medicine. Am Coll Cardiol 2018;. https://www.acc.org/latest-in-cardiology/articles/2018/01/04/12/42/cover-story-digital-health-solutions-in-cardiovascular-medicine. Accessed March 21, 2022.

11. Covid-19 United States cases by county. Johns Hopkins Coronavirus resource center. Available at: https://coronavirus.jhu.edu/us-map. Accessed March 21, 2022.

12. Rogers Everett M. Diffusion of innovations. New York: Free Press; 1995. Print.

13. Guo C, Ashrafian H, Ghafur S, et al. Challenges for the evaluation of digital health solutions—a call for innovative evidence generation approaches. NPJ digital Med 2020;3(1):1–14.

14. Lalla-Edward ST, Mashabane N, Stewart-Isherwood L, et al. Implementation of an mHealth app to promote engagement during HIV care and viral load suppression in Johannesburg, South Africa (iThemba life): pilot Technical feasibility and acceptability study. JMIR Formative Res 2022;6(2):e26033.

15. Digital health market size & growth report, 2021-2028. Available at: https://www.grandviewresearch.com/industry-analysis/digital-health-market#:~:text=The%20global%20digital%20health%20market,15.1%25%20from%202021%20to%202028. Accessed March 28, 2022.

16. Reyzelman AM, Koelewyn K, Murphy M, et al. Continuous temperature-monitoring socks for home Use in patients with diabetes: observational study. J Med Internet Res 2018;20(12):e12460.

17. High utilization telepodiatry for diabetic foot management. Siren. https://www.siren.care/for-providers. Accessed March 29, 2022.

18. Siren socks provider Stories. Siren. Available at: https://www.siren.care/provider-stories. Accessed March 29, 2022.

19. Zhong A, Li G, Wang D, et al. The risks and external effects of diabetic foot ulcer on diabetic patients: a hospital-based survey in Wuhan area, China. Wound Repair Regen 2017;25(5):858–63.

20. Type 2 diabetes. Centers for disease control and prevention. 2021. Available at: https://www.cdc.gov/diabetes/basics/type2.html. Accessed March 31, 2022.

21. Stein N, Brooks K. A fully automated conversational artificial intelligence for weight loss: longitudinal observational study among Overweight and obese Adults. JMIR Diabetes 2017;2(2):e28.
22. Expanding rpm across Riley hospital for Children. Locus health. Available at: https://www.locushealth.com/case-study/riley-hospital-for-children/. Accessed March 29, 2022.
23. Our network - NPC-QIC. NPC. Available at: https://npc-qic.squarespace.com/our-network/#success. Accessed March 29, 2022.
24. She has a heart baby at home and the Riley Team "in her back pocket". Riley Children's Health. https://www.rileychildrens.org/connections/she-has-a-heart-baby-at-home-and-the-riley-team-in-her-back-pocket. Accessed March 29, 2022.
25. Contributor Messler J. CMS has decided to put its muscle behind glycemic management-why now? AJMC. 2021. Available at: https://www.ajmc.com/view/contributor-cms-has-decided-to-put-its-muscle-behind-glycemic-management-why-now-. Accessed February 29, 2022.
26. Pierson E, Cutler DM, Leskovec J, et al. An algorithmic approach to reducing unexplained pain disparities in underserved populations. Nat Med 2021;27(1):136–40.
27. Wearable medical devices market size report, 2021-2028. 2021. Available at: https://www.grandviewresearch.com/industry-analysis/wearable-medical-devices-marke.t. Accessed March 29, 2022.
28. Driscoll A. Glytec and Roche announce strategic partnership to bring Digital Health Innovation in glycemic decision support to the hospital bedside. Image. 2022. Available at: https://glytecsystems.com/news/glytec-and-roche-announce-strategic-partnership-to-bring-digital-health-innovation-in-glycemic-decision-support-to-the-hospital-bedside/. Accessed March 29, 2022.
29. Eberly L, Richter D, Comerci G, et al. Psychosocial and demographic factors influencing pain scores of patients with knee osteoarthritis. PLOS ONE 2018;13(4):e0195075.
30. Cancer key Facts. World health organization. Available at: https://www.who.int/news-room/fact-sheets/detail/cancer. Accessed March 21, 2022.
31. Tumor boards-what are they and how can they help you? Cancer Commons. 2021. Available at: https://cancercommons.org/latest-insights/cancer-tumor-boards-how-they-help-patients/. Accessed March 21, 2022.
32. Hammer RD, Prime MS. A clinician's perspective on co-developing and co-implementing a digital tumor board solution. Health Informatics J 2020;26(3):2213–21.
33. Krupinski E, Comas M, Gallego L. A new software platform to improve multidisciplinary tumor board workflows and user satisfaction: a pilot study. J Pathol Inform 2018;9(1):9–26.
34. Hammer RD, Fowler D, Sheets LR, et al. Digital tumor board solutions have significant impact on case preparation. JCO Clin Cancer Inform 2020;(4):757–68.
35. Golda N. Setting our sights on the right target: how addressing physician burnout may be a solution for improved patient experience. Clin Dermatol 2019;37(6):685–8.
36. Lichtner V, Baysari M. Electronic display of a patient treatment over time: a perspective on clinicians' burn-out. BMJ Health Care Inform 2021;28(1):e100281.

Opportunities and Challenges with Artificial Intelligence in Genomics

Danielle E. Kurant, MD

KEYWORDS

- Artificial intelligence • Machine learning • Genomics

KEY POINTS

- Artificial intelligence (AI) algorithms applied to genomic data can detect cancer, classify variants, and predict gene expression, among many other applications.
- Historical inequities and biases exist in current, predominantly European-based data sets, which may lead to further inequities. "Fair" algorithms are being developed to address this.
- Models developed from datasets of predominantly European ancestry may not translate well into other populations; therefore, diverse data sets are required.
- There are ethical and legal considerations when building algorithms based on sensitive genomic data, and care must be taken to implement these models responsibly.

BACKGROUND

Artificial intelligence (AI) and machine learning (ML) have drastically changed society since their inception. This technology permeates every industry from targeted advertising to approval for credit cards and loans and even plays a role in aspects of the health care industry. The study of the human genome has likewise had a major impact on society, both in the hospital setting and even with commercially available genetic tests for ancestry and certain cancer risk genes. Both AI and genomic medicine are centered around data and have been made possible by advances in technology. It is perhaps, therefore, unsurprising that they synergize so well for the advancement of scientific knowledge and the diagnosis and management of patients. Here the authors explore a selection of topics in which AI has been used and/or has the opportunity to advance genomic medicine. Current and future challenges are also discussed, including algorithmic fairness, data security and privacy, and interpretability.

Medical Oncology, Dana-Farber Cancer Institute, Harvard Medical School, Boston, MA, USA
E-mail address: danielle_kurant@dfci.harvard.edu

Clin Lab Med 43 (2023) 87–97
https://doi.org/10.1016/j.cll.2022.09.007
labmed.theclinics.com

VARIANTS OF UNCERTAIN SIGNIFICANCE

All individuals will have numerous single nucleotide variants (SNVs) in protein coding regions of their genomes as compared with others or to a reference human genome sequence. However, many such variants, particularly those that are rare, will be variants of uncertain significance (VUS). By definition, VUS are neither known to have a phenotypic impact nor known to not have one (and if they do have an impact, the nature of the impact is uncertain). VUS comprise the vast majority of SNVs identified in any patient genomic or exomic analysis.

A typical workflow in the clinical evaluation of patient genomic testing involves algorithmic identification of variants from sequencing data followed by manual review of online databases such as ClinVar, OMIM, and ClinGen, among other resources. Literature is reviewed for reports and interpretations of the variants in question, and the variant is then deemed to be pathogenic, benign, or of uncertain significance. Guidelines have been published by the American College of Medical Genetics and Genomics (ACMG) and the Association for Molecular Pathology (AMP) regarding the interpretation of these variants.[1] VUS pose a particular challenge to clinicians, and often the interpretation of these variants changes as new data are uncovered. As a classification question in a large and complex data set, this is an excellent application for AI-based approaches.[2] To that end, many algorithms have been developed that predict the deleteriousness of variants based on biophysical properties, such as PolyPhen-2,[3] SIFT,[4] and PROVEAN.[5]

The categorization of VUS can be achieved via supervised or unsupervised methods. Using supervised methods of machine learning, labels come from manually curated mutations and/or experiments. Unsupervised methods, however, allow for the development of classification models from unlabeled data by learning some underlying structure within the data points or integrating external information. Several supervised methods using AI/ML have been developed to determine the likelihood of a variant being deleterious. DEOGEN2, for example, incorporates information about the molecular effects, involved domains, gene relevance, and gene interactions. This information is then "mapped" into a deleteriousness score for the variant. This tool is a predictor for missense SNVs for human proteins. It uses evolutionary-based features, prediction of early folding protein residues, features related to protein domains, interaction patches, and gene- and pathway-oriented features. This model achieved comparable performance with other published predictors in the **Humsavar16** dataset.[6]

High-throughput experiments have been developed that can evaluate thousands of variants simultaneously, called multiplexed assays of variant effects.[7,8] These high-throughput sequencing assays interrogate the effects of various variant types and allow for massive scalability of functional assays.[9] Historically, most functional assays have been reactive, wherein a variant will surface clinically, then a functional assay will be performed to explore the effects of the variant. However, given the vast number of uncharacterized variants that exist, and with current computing power that is available, it becomes attractive to take a more proactive experimental approach. Evolutionary model of variant effect (EVE) is an example of unsupervised learning in the classification of variants. EVE classifies human genetic variants solely on evolutionary sequences, looking at the distribution of sequence variation across different species to determine the likelihood of pathogenicity in humans. The model outperforms other state-of-the-art computational methods of variant classification. In fact, EVE has been found to be as accurate as high-throughput experiments in variant classification. The model was able to predict the pathogenicity of more than 36 million variants, including evidence for the classification of more than 256,000 VUS.[10]

POLYGENIC RISK SCORES

In addition to classifying VUS, the integration of genomics and AI has many applications in the diagnosis and management of disease risk. To improve patient outcomes, it is essential to identify disease and disease risk as early as possible in order to initiate interventions at the appropriate time. Historically, the search for genetic risk for disease has focused on rare monogenic variants; however, a large fraction of disease risk is explained by common variants and is highly polygenic (involving hundreds or thousands of genes)[11]; this presents several problems: first, how does one combine the effects of many variants across the genome to make a helpful prediction? Second, how would this model combine with other existing clinical data and tools? And finally, how should the uncertainty of a given score be quantified[12]?

A polygenic risk score (PRS) is a calculated risk summary that an individual will develop a specific phenotype. These scores evaluate common genetic variants across the genome for a variety of phenotypes. A computational algorithm is then applied to combine these data into a single number that serves as a summary for an individual's inherited susceptibility to the phenotype. Although various conditions have known driver mutations, many diseases are polygenic, affected by genetic variants across the human genome. Genome-wide association studies (GWAS) have identified thousands of genetic differences between individuals who develop certain diseases and those who do not; however, each individual variant's contribution may be negligible. A PRS allows for the summation of these miniscule risks across the genome that, when combined, provide useful information about individual's susceptibility to certain inherited conditions.[11,13,14]

One challenge in integrating these scores into the clinical workflow is that the correlation between true risk and inferred risk tends to be highest in the population from which GWAS statistics were derived. Both the frequency and correlation of genetic variants can vary substantially among different ancestries,[15] and it is well demonstrated that PRSs built on datasets of predominantly European ancestry do not translate well into other groups.[14,16] As many available datasets are mainly composed of individuals of European ancestry, this can cause issues with transferability of models into other populations. Scores inferred from European GWASs (such as with 1000 Genomes Project reference panel) are susceptible to biases in any direction and as such have limited transferability to other populations. Generalized risk prediction methods and increased diversity within reference panels are essential for development of PRSs that will benefit people from various backgrounds[17] and are an active area of ML research.

Early identification of individuals at high risk for certain clinical conditions is crucial for appropriate screening and targeted prevention and treatment strategies. Although existing clinical models serve to identify a group of "high-risk" individuals, there are still those who do not meet these criteria yet are at higher genetic risk than the general population. One example of this is cardiac disease, where a neural network–based risk model using both clinical and polygenic predictors has been deployed in patients from the UK Biobank.[16] PRSs were combined with clinical information to identify a population of patients at low to intermediate clinical risk who were at increased overall risk for a major adverse cardiac event within 10 years. Such integrative models have the potential to reduce population disease burden and even improve patient outcomes by allowing for early intervention. PRSs use hundreds of thousands of single nucleotide polymorphisms to predict phenotypes. These scores are strong predictors for risk and may combine well with existing risk scores to generate useful clinical models.[18] Several groups have looked at adding PRSs to existing models. Although there have been mixed results, the addition of PRSs to clinical data has been shown to improve discrimination and reclassification. PRSs have the potential to aid in the identification of high-genetic-risk individuals, allowing health care providers to intervene before patients develop the phenotype of an adverse event.[16]

Another application of PRSs is the evaluation of individual risk for treatment response or toxicity. Some patients, for example, develop immune-related adverse events secondary to treatment with immune checkpoint inhibitors. Because there is significant variation among individuals with regard to tumor response and immune toxicity from these treatments, the ability to anticipate patient response may contribute to improved patient safety and outcomes. A PRS derived from a hypothyroidism GWAS demonstrated that lifetime risk for autoimmune thyroid disease is also informative for risk of developing a thyroid immune-related adverse event during treatment with atezolizumab. This PRS was also associated with lower risk of death in patients with triple-negative breast cancer, demonstrating a role for PRS in the guidance of cancer immunotherapy in clinical management.[19] However, the application of PRS to treatment outcomes is still in its clinical infancy, and further studies are needed to determine the most effective way to bring this into clinical practice. A key consideration in these individual risk assessments is the estimation of uncertainty. Whether or not a variant is causal and the presence of statistical noise both contribute to the uncertainty of a PRS. Most assessments of PRS accuracy have been at the cohort level in studies; however, it is also important to gauge the individual accuracy, as computational algorithms will likely be used on individual patients. Uncertainty is also relevant at the patient level as nongenetic factors also contribute to the individual's overall risk for a specific phenotype.[12]

GENETIC ANCESTRY AND RELATEDNESS

GWAS have allowed for advances in mapping complex traits in groups of ostensibly unrelated individuals. These same studies, however, have revealed hidden relatedness among individuals in publicly available databases even after accounting for population-scale ancestry. Relatedness becomes a relevant issue to tackle when considering building models based on these datasets. When models are trained on large populations of purported unrelated individuals, it becomes essential to identify and account for hidden relatedness, as relatedness can bias associations in the shared regions of their genomes in addition to population statistics. Various approaches have been developed to quantify relatedness, such as genome-wide estimates[20] and segment-by-segment analysis.[21] However, these methods can be computationally expensive, and as larger data sets are generated their use becomes impractical.[22]

Gusev and colleagues developed GERMLINE (genetic error-tolerant regional matching with linear-time extension), an algorithm for identifying individual segments of recent common ancestry between individuals. The algorithm, based on a dictionary of haplotypes, rapidly identified portions of the genome that were identical and then expanded these segments to longer, probabilistically similar segments.[23] The algorithm was benchmarked using both real and simulated data. GERMLINE had a higher sensitivity and lower overall false-positive rate than PLINK in simulated data and ran greater than 100x faster than PLINK.[22,24] Recently, this approach has been further improved on with iLASH (Identical By Descent by LocAlity-Sensitive Hashing), which instead directly identifies short *approximately* identical segments among individuals. This more efficient method can search through hundreds of thousands of individuals for genetic matches quickly.[24]

One area in which ancestry-based solutions are beneficial is transcriptome-wide association studies (TWAS). Integrating both GWAS and gene expression data into TWAS may better elucidate disease mechanisms. As with other data sets, it is essential to include data from multiple genetic ancestries to generate prediction models that are transferrable to other populations. Multiancestry transcriptome-wide analysis (METRO) has been presented as a method that can use gene expression data from multiple genetic ancestries to improve TWAS. Most existing TWAS methods focus on expression studies from a single genetic ancestry. The METRO method, however, uses expression data from multiple ancestries, using a joint likelihood-based inference framework.[25]

CANCER

In combination with AI, genomics has many applications to cancer detection, diagnosis, and treatment, including both genomic profiling of tumors to inform therapy selection and "liquid biopsies." Liquid biopsies seek to detect cancer by sequencing circulating DNA in patients before the onset of clinical symptoms. Cell-free DNA (cfDNA) is fragmented DNA released in body fluids from the apoptosis or necrosis of cells. When cfDNA comes from cancer cells, it is referred to as circulating tumor DNA (ctDNA). These ctDNA fragments have been used for the detection of somatic mutations in patients with cancer, disease monitoring, and even therapy guidance.[26] However, the low signal-to-noise ratio in addition to tumor heterogeneity poses a challenge for the use of naïve ctDNA measurements for clinical care. It may be possible to detect mutations from various clones in heterogeneous tumors using liquid biopsy; however, tumor heterogeneity drives down the expected tumor fraction of any somatic variants that may be detected in ctDNA: a sample that already contains a miniscule amount of genetic material. Moreover, it is also essential to be able to pinpoint tumor location and ideally to estimate tumor fraction. Challenges in detection such as these can be overcome using AI-based methods.

Thus far, cfDNA has typically been used for the detection of somatic SNVs. There have been attempts to detect copy number alterations in ctDNA; however, the low signal-to-noise ratio makes it difficult to differentiate these from noise in the sample. Deep learning may serve as an effective method for cancer detection in plasma donors, showing high accuracy with hepatocellular carcinoma detection in one study.[27] Deep learning has been used to assess both the DNA sequence and methylation state of reads in plasma donors to predict the risk that the donor has cancer. DISMIR (Deep learning–based noninvasive cancer detection by integrating DNA sequence and methylation information of individual cell-free DNA reads) predicted the likelihood that a given sequencing read was derived from cancer tissue and assigned it a score based on its DNA sequence and methylation state. These scores were then integrated into an overall cancer risk prediction.[27] Tools such as CancerLocator go one step further, not merely detecting the presence of a tumor but also predicting its location. Methylation is known to vary between cancer and normal cells and can thus serve as a target for cell of origin detection from liquid biopsies.[28,29] CancerLocator uses methylation data to infer both tumor fraction and tissue of origin from ctDNA.[30] The fraction of ctDNA in cfDNA has been shown to correlate with tumor burden[31]; this is significant, as tumor burden can have clinical implications including prognosis, therapeutic efficacy, and likelihood of cytokine release syndrome.[32,33]

Another application of AI and ML to cancer is the determination of whether a cancer is the result of inherited germline mutations or a cancer predisposition syndrome. This distinction can affect patient treatment and prognosis and is essential for counseling patients and family members about their risks. Traditionally, paired tumor and normal sequencing has been used to identify germline variants that may be contributing to the patient's presentation. In the clinical setting, genetic panels targeted to the most common cancer drivers are typically used, including MSK-IMPACT (Memorial Sloan Kettering-Integrated Mutation Profiling of Actionable Cancer Targets), Foundation Medicine, and Tempus. In one study, MSK-IMPACT identified all germline variants in patient DNA samples tested, in addition to additional pathogenic mutations in 16 of those samples. However, existing tumor panels still fail to capture all drivers at low cost.[34]

AI may provide an alternative approach to developing targeted sequencing panels. In one study, ML was used to guide the development of a targeted sequencing panel that identified top candidate mutations in known driver genes and transcription factor binding sites related to prostate cancer.[35] Whole genome sequencing data were captured from prostate tumors to develop a targeted panel of indels that was then screened in silico in prostate tumor sequences from patients. The panel was then tested using prospectively collected cfDNA and tumor from a set of patients with prostate cancer. The team generated a targeted sequencing panel that focused on coding and regulatory noncoding regions that could potentially be sites of deleterious mutations. The panel was able to detect tumor variants in the cfDNA of all patients from the test set.[35]

Certain mutations can signify the increase of resistance of tumors to treatments. The timely and accurate identification of these resistance mutations is essential for optimizing patient management and outcomes. This process can be predicted using AI, as demonstrated by the development of the pathway-aware multilayered hierarchical network (P-NET). P-NET is a biologically informed deep learning model, where the structure of the learning model is itself defined using prior biological knowledge. More than 3000 curated biological pathways were used to create a neural network into which molecular profiles of individuals could be passed. These data were then distributed into nodes representing sets of genes. This model focused on mutations and copy-number alterations. Candidate genes were validated to elucidate their function and their mechanism of action. The trained network outperformed other models including decision trees, logistic regression, and support vector machines, with a smaller sample size. The generation of a biologically informed model allowed for the use of a smaller number of parameters, thus allowing for greater interpretability of the model. The importance of interpretable models is discussed later in this article. P-NET predicted advanced prostate disease based on genomic profile, in addition to potential biochemical recurrence. P-NET also accurately classified castration-resistant metastatic versus primary prostate cancers.[36]

OUTSTANDING ISSUES

As large-scale datasets with molecular indicators of disease have been generated and interrogated, the need for algorithms that can learn from these data has increased. However, numerous challenges remain. Some of the challenges are technical in nature, including insufficient interoperability of clinical genomic data. Other challenges go beyond the technical realm to include ethical and legal considerations. These include addressing historical inequities (which continue to affect our ability to fully and optimally apply genomic technologies across diverse groups of patients) and also addressing important risks to patient privacy. These challenges remain largely unresolved in the clinical use of these technologies.

HISTORICAL INEQUITIES

One major issue with the use of AI in data sets such as these is the possibility of perpetuating or even worsening existing health disparities. In many cases, algorithms are learning from decisions or classifications that have historically been made based on biases against specific populations. When models are built from these historical prejudices, there is substantial risk of perpetuating or worsening inequities and biases. Work is being done to develop models and modeling methods that account for this issue.

When developing algorithms, it is essential to remember that they will be in use in the real world. Although overall prediction accuracy is important, great lengths must be taken to ensure that the outcome of a model will not unfairly prevent someone from accessing needed care or resources, and the societal impact of algorithmic decisions must be considered. Addressing causality is essential to the work of designing fair algorithms. The definition of "fairness" is also relevant, as, depending on the attribute in question, it is possible to increase inequity with certain definitions of "fairness." The concept of "counterfactual fairness" relates to the idea that an algorithmic decision is considered fair if it is the same in the real world and also in a "counterfactual world" in which the individual belongs to a different demographic. In other words, a distribution of possible predictions for an individual should be the same in a world where the protected attributes in the model were different. Although the technical details of counterfactual fairness are outside the scope of this paper, the concept of fairness is essential to the development of any clinical algorithm.[37] In genomics, this may have implications in treatment selection, access to clinical trials, or other clinically relevant decisions.

PRIVACY

Another consideration when working with genomic data is the sensitive nature of the data. Information contained in an individual's genetic code has implications for both the individual themselves and the individual's relatives, and this brings up complex considerations regarding the nature of consent, as testing and decisions made based on one consented individual's genetics may have the potential to affect other genetically related individuals who were not consented. Moreover, studies that identify populations of individuals have the potential to affect individuals who were neither consented nor tested themselves. One example of this was a GWAS study investigating the genetics of same-sex sexual behavior.[38] Concern was raised about the ethics and motivation behind such a study, which despite exploring a topic of potential interest to biologists (nonreproductive sexual behavior in animals), also explored the genetics behind an already at-risk population.[39]

Relevant privacy regulations have been passed, such as the General Data Protection Regulation (GDPR). The GDPR delineates regulations for the collection, storage, and usage of personal information. The GDPR requires that an individual should have the right not to be subject to a decision based solely on automated processing, such as profiling related to health. Any automated profiling should prevent discriminatory effects based on factors such as race or ethnicity. Per Article 9, data processing involving health data is disallowed, with relevant exceptions in cases of explicit consent or when processing is "necessary for the purposes of preventive or occupational medicine" or for medical diagnosis.[40] Although it is unclear exactly how this will apply to genomic AI/ML-based tools, privacy law will certainly play a role in the development and application of these models globally. The GDPR requires explicit informed consent for the collection of personal information. Although informed consent is already used for medical procedures, it may be difficult to obtain truly informed consent for AI-driven care decisions. Moreover, the GDPR requirement for right to explanation may limit the types of models that can be used in clinical tools.[41]

One potential approach to maintaining patient privacy while training models is federated learning. Although standard machine learning approaches train models on centralized training data, federated learning allows for the development of a shared model while keeping data stored at separate remote locations. With federated learning, a central model can be downloaded, then updated with local data, and then the update sent to a central server. There the local updates can be aggregated into one unified global model[42]; this prevents the need for storage or transfer of sensitive data across the Internet. In addition, protocols exist that protect individual privacy by only decrypting the average updates when a large number of models has been aggregated. Google has introduced this approach as a means of aggregating high-dimensional data for models from mobile phone users in a secure manner, and a similar approach could potentially be used for aggregating information from individuals or health care organizations.[43]

EXPLAINABILITY

Both GDPR requirements for explainability of models and clinician hesitancy to adopt complex models can be barriers to the implementation of AI/ML algorithms in clinical practice. Explainable models can help give decision-makers and stakeholders confidence in including AI-based tools in clinical practice. With supervised learning, the quality of the models developed is contingent on the quality of the initial labels used to train the algorithm. The ability of a model's reasoning to be explained and/or understood by a human operator ostensibly allows for a clinician to perform a logic check of sorts. In this setting, a human clinician could look at the reasoning of a model and determine whether it is clinically sound, thereby giving confidence that the output of the model in question is also sound/reliable.[44] Explainable algorithms may also be helpful for reducing bias, thereby further protecting patients who may be subject to clinical decisions based on these models. Some tools have already included features to assist in understanding algorithmic decisions. HistoMapr-Breast, for example, has clickable button that displays why the region of interest was classified as it was. Similar easily accessible explanations can and should be included in current and future AI/ML-based tools in order to encourage clinician confidence and protect patients.[44]

SUMMARY

Advances in AI and ML offer great promise in the field of genomics. The utility of these technologies has already been demonstrated in several areas, with more applications being explored and developed. However, the sensitive nature of genomic data, in addition to the potential for perpetuating or worsening health disparities, means the development of these models must be approached with great care. It is essential to protect vulnerable individuals and populations and to ensure patient privacy when handling sensitive genetic information. Diverse data sets and interpretable models can help to develop fair, explainable algorithms that can be broadly applied across ancestries.

DISCLOSURE

The author has nothing to disclose.

ACKNOWLEDGMENTS

The author would like to thank Alexander Gusev, Jason Baron, and the members of Gusev Lab for their helpful conversations and insights regarding the topics covered in this article. D E. Kurant was supported by grant R01CA244569.

REFERENCES

1. Richards S, Aziz N, Bale S, et al. Standards and guidelines for the interpretation of sequence variants: a joint consensus recommendation of the American College of medical genetics and genomics and the association for molecular Pathology. Genet Med 2015;17(5):405–24.
2. Dong C, Wei P, Jian X, et al. Comparison and integration of deleteriousness prediction methods for nonsynonymous SNVs in whole exome sequencing studies. Hum Mol Genet 2015;24(8):2125–37.
3. Adzhubei I, Jordan DM, Sunyaev SR. Predicting functional effect of human missense mutations using PolyPhen-2. Curr Protoc Hum Genet 2013. https://doi.org/10.1002/0471142905.hg0720s76. Chapter 7:Unit7 20.
4. Ng PC, Henikoff S. Predicting deleterious amino acid substitutions. Genome Res 2001;11(5):863–74.
5. Choi Y, Sims GE, Murphy S, et al. Predicting the functional effect of amino acid substitutions and indels. PLoS One 2012;7(10):e46688.
6. Raimondi D, Tanyalcin I, Ferté J, et al. DEOGEN2: prediction and interactive visualization of single amino acid variant deleteriousness in human proteins. Nucleic Acids Res 2017;45(W1):W201–6.
7. Esposito D, Weile J, Shendure J, et al. MaveDB: an open-source platform to distribute and interpret data from multiplexed assays of variant effect. Genome Biol 2019;20(1):223.
8. Trenkmann M. Putting genetic variants to a fitness test. Nat Rev Genet 2018; 19(11):667.
9. Weile J, Roth FP. Multiplexed assays of variant effects contribute to a growing genotype-phenotype atlas. Hum Genet 2018;137(9):665–78.
10. Frazer J, Notin P, Dias M, et al. Disease variant prediction with deep generative models of evolutionary data. Nature 2021;599(7883):91–5.
11. Khera AV, Chaffin M, Aragam KG, et al. Genome-wide polygenic scores for common diseases identify individuals with risk equivalent to monogenic mutations. Nat Genet 2018;50(9):1219–24.
12. Ding Y, Hou K, Burch KS, et al. Large uncertainty in individual polygenic risk score estimation impacts PRS-based risk stratification. Nat Genet 2022; 54(1):30–9.
13. Läll K, Mägi R, Morris A, et al. Personalized risk prediction for type 2 diabetes: the potential of genetic risk scores. Genet Med 2017;19(3):322–9.
14. Martin AR, Kanai M, Kamatani Y, et al. Clinical use of current polygenic risk scores may exacerbate health disparities. Nat Genet 2019;51(4):584–91.
15. Carrot-Zhang J, Chambwe N, Damrauer JS, et al. Comprehensive analysis of genetic ancestry and its molecular correlates in cancer. Cancer Cell 2020;37(5): 639–54.e6.
16. Steinfeldt J, Buergel T, Loock L, et al. Neural network-based integration of polygenic and clinical information: development and validation of a prediction model for 10-year risk of major adverse cardiac events in the UK Biobank cohort. Lancet Digital Health 2022;4(2):e84–94.

17. Martin AR, Gignoux CR, Walters RK, et al. Human Demographic history impacts genetic risk prediction across diverse populations. Am J Hum Genet 2017;100(4): 635–49.
18. Figtree GA, Vernon ST, Nicholls SJ. Taking the next steps to implement polygenic risk scoring for improved risk stratification and primary prevention of coronary artery disease. Eur J Prev Cardiol 2020;29(4):580–7.
19. Khan Z, Hammer C, Carroll J, et al. Genetic variation associated with thyroid autoimmunity shapes the systemic immune response to PD-1 checkpoint blockade. Nat Commun 2021;12(1):3355.
20. Mao Y, Xu S. A Monte Carlo algorithm for computing the IBD matrices using incomplete marker information. Heredity (Edinb) 2005;94(3):305–15.
21. Hill WG, Hernández-Sánchez J. Prediction of multilocus identity-by-descent. Genetics 2007;176(4):2307–15.
22. Gusev A, Lowe JK, Stoffel M, et al. Whole population, genome-wide mapping of hidden relatedness. Genome Res 2009;19(2):318–26.
23. Purcell S, Neale B, Todd-Brown K, et al. PLINK: a tool set for whole-genome association and population-based linkage analyses. Am J Hum Genet 2007;81(3): 559–75.
24. Shemirani R, Belbin GM, Avery CL, et al. Rapid detection of identity-by-descent tracts for mega-scale datasets. Nat Commun 2021;12(1):3546.
25. Li Z, Zhao W, Shang L, et al. METRO: multi-ancestry transcriptome-wide association studies for powerful gene-trait association detection. Am J Hum Genet 2022;109(5):783–801.
26. Powles T, Assaf ZJ, Davarpanah N, et al. ctDNA guiding adjuvant immunotherapy in urothelial carcinoma. Nature 2021;595(7867):432–7.
27. Li J, Wei L, Zhang X, et al. DISMIR: deep learning-based noninvasive cancer detection by integrating DNA sequence and methylation information of individual cell-free DNA reads. Brief Bioinform 2021;22(6). https://doi.org/10.1093/bib/bbab250.
28. Feinberg AP, Ohlsson R, Henikoff S. The epigenetic progenitor origin of human cancer. Nat Rev Genet 2006;7(1):21–33.
29. Alvarez H, Opalinska J, Zhou L, et al. Widespread hypomethylation occurs early and synergizes with gene amplification during esophageal carcinogenesis. PLoS Genet 2011;7(3):e1001356.
30. Kang S, Li Q, Chen Q, et al. CancerLocator: non-invasive cancer diagnosis and tissue-of-origin prediction using methylation profiles of cell-free DNA. Genome Biol 2017;18(1):53.
31. Adalsteinsson VA, Ha G, Freeman SS, et al. Scalable whole-exome sequencing of cell-free DNA reveals high concordance with metastatic tumors. Nat Commun 2017;8(1):1324.
32. Czarnecka AM, Brodziak A, Sobczuk P, et al. Metastatic tumor burden and loci as predictors of first line sunitinib treatment efficacy in patients with renal cell carcinoma. Sci Rep 2019;9(1):7754.
33. Li M, Xue S-L, Tang X, et al. The differential effects of tumor burdens on predicting the net benefits of ssCART-19 cell treatment on r/r B-ALL patients. Sci Rep 2022; 12(1):378.
34. Cheng DT, Prasad M, Chekaluk Y, et al. Comprehensive detection of germline variants by MSK-IMPACT, a clinical diagnostic platform for solid tumor molecular oncology and concurrent cancer predisposition testing. BMC Med Genomics 2017;10(1):33.

35. Cario CL, Chen E, Leong L, et al. A machine learning approach to optimizing cell-free DNA sequencing panels: with an application to prostate cancer. BMC Cancer 2020;20(1):820.
36. Elmarakeby HA, Hwang J, Arafeh R, et al. Biologically informed deep neural network for prostate cancer discovery. Nature 2021/10/01 2021;598(7880): 348–52.
37. Kusner MJ, Loftus J, Russell C, et al. Counterfactual fairness. Adv Neural Inf Process Syst 2017;30.
38. Ganna A, Verweij Karin JH, Nivard Michel G, et al. Large-scale GWAS reveals insights into the genetic architecture of same-sex sexual behavior. Science 2019; 365(6456):eaat7693.
39. Vitti J. Opinion: big data scientists must be ethicists too. 2019. https://www.broadinstitute.org/blog/opinion-big-data-scientists-must-be-ethicists-too. [Accessed 28 June 2022].
40. European Parliament, Council of the European Union. Regulation (EU) 2016/679 of the European Parliament and of the Council of 27 April 2016 on the protection of natural persons with regard to the processing of personal data and on the free movement of such data, and repealing Directive 95/46/EC (General Data Protection Regulation). Official Journal of the European Union 2016;59(L 119):1–88. http://data.europa.eu/eli/reg/2016/679/oj. [Accessed 14 October 2022].
41. He J, Baxter SL, Xu J, et al. The practical implementation of artificial intelligence technologies in medicine. Nat Med 2019;25(1):30–6.
42. Konečný J., McMahan H.B., Yu F.X., et al., Federated learning: Strategies for improving communication efficiency, 2016. Available at: https://research.google/pubs/pub45648/. Accessed 10 May 2022.
43. McMahan B, Ramage D. Federated learning: collaborative machine learning without centralized training data 2017. Available at: https://ai.googleblog.com/2017/04/federated-learning-collaborative.html. [Accessed 28 June 2022].
44. Tosun AB, Pullara F, Becich MJ, et al. Explainable AI (xAI) for Anatomic Pathology. Adv Anat Pathol 2020;27(4):241–50.

Using Artificial Intelligence to Better Predict and Develop Biomarkers

Sam A. Michelhaugh, BA[a,1], James L. Januzzi Jr, MD[b,c,d,*]

KEYWORDS

- Genomics • Transcriptomics • Proteomics • Metabolomics • Artificial intelligence
- Biomarkers • Heart failure

KEY POINTS

- Biomarker discovery has been enhanced by the high-throughput technologies of omics.
- Artificial intelligence improves statistical analysis of the large data sets generated in omics to enhance identification of markers of potential interest.
- Application of omics, especially proteomics, has aided with identification of biomarkers with clinical relevance to heart failure.
- Through biomarker discovery, researchers can further study identified biomarkers to determine clinical utility, pathophysiology, and improve patient care.

INTRODUCTION

Given the complex pathophysiology and etiologies of heart failure (HF), tailoring care to improve patient outcomes and quality of life involves the integration of multiple parameters.[1] Beyond adjusting treatments based on symptoms and physical examination findings, clinicians must rely on adjunctive testing to support their judgment; this includes imaging and measurement of circulating biomarkers. Most notably, among biomarkers measured, natriuretic peptides are considered the standard of care for treating patients with HF.[2,3] However, HF is a complicated condition, which cannot be summarized by one biomarker alone.[4,5] Although natriuretic peptides indicate cardiomyocyte stretch, they have limited ability to capture other changes associated with HF remodeling included inflammation, oxidative stress, and fibrosis.[6,7]

This article originally appeared in *Heart Failure Clinics*, Volume 18 Issue 2, April 2022.
a Georgetown University School of Medicine, Washington, DC, USA; b Department of Medicine, Division of Cardiology, Massachusetts General Hospital, 55 Fruit Street, Boston, MA 02114, USA; c Department of Medicine, Division of Cardiology, Harvard Medical School, Boston, MA, USA; d Baim Institute for Clinical Research, Boston, MA, USA
1 2500 Wisconsin Avenue Northwest, APT 948, Washington, DC 20007.
* Corresponding author.
E-mail address: jjanuzzi@partners.org

Clin Lab Med 43 (2023) 99–114
https://doi.org/10.1016/j.cll.2022.09.021
labmed.theclinics.com

For this reason, multiple markers are needed to recognize the pathophysiology of HF and tailor care to optimize patient outcomes.

The introduction of omics, including genomics, transcriptomics, proteomics, and metabolomics, has enhanced biomarker discovery.[8–11] Omics allows for analysis of biological pathways involved in aspects of the central dogma and biological modifications of products. Using high-throughput and untargeted omics technologies provides better phenotyping and unveils previously unknown HF pathophysiology. Furthermore, integration of findings of multiple omics studies gives a comprehensive understanding of pathophysiology from the level of genes to final metabolites to recognize where disease processes arise.[12–14] Discovery of markers enables researchers and clinicians to recognize potential risks for developing HF, serve as prognostic indicators, or ascertain druggable targets for future therapeutic interventions.[15]

BACKGROUND

Previous work in biomarker research involved the testing of suspected markers individually. Through this process, individual markers were selected from proposed biological processes or previous research results. This hypothesis-driven process is inefficient and costly in terms of money, time, and sample used for each experiment.[16] With the advent of omics, experimenters can test multiple markers simultaneously.[12–14] Beyond improving throughput and decreasing waste, omics reduces bias as it is inductive, and allows for the identification of markers that may have otherwise not been considered.[17,18]

Modern omics technologies have great potential for researchers to improve efficiencies. In individual experiments, it is possible to test hundreds to thousands of individual targets simultaneously while using as little as 1 μL of sample or using a single cell.[19–21] Omics experiments are also being aided by technological advancements. Previous analysis would involve intensive statistics to sort through large data sets to identify markers of interest. Use of artificial intelligence (AI) in analysis makes result interpretation easier, faster, and more feasible for researchers who do not have access to biostatisticians capable of analyzing such data (**Fig. 1**).[12–14,22–24] We will discuss the broad range of omics possibilities but then focus on the area of proteomics.

THE OMICS MULTIVERSE
Genomics

In contrast to genetics (the study of heredity), genomics is the study of the entirety of all deoxyribonucleic acid (DNA) within an organism (**Fig. 2**). In certain diseases with underlying genetic components, understanding the genome helps identify patients at risk for developing particular diseases. With improved DNA sequencing technologies, the genome can be characterized through genome-wide association studies (GWASs). GWAS aims to identify variations in genes, such as single nucleotide polymorphisms, a substitution of an individual DNA base in the sequence.[12,13,25] Genomics in HF research has unveiled new insights into HF pathophysiology, such as identification of 2 loci where single nucleotide polymorphisms may predict future development of HF.[26–28]

Original DNA sequencing relied on the Sanger method, whereas newer and more efficient processes for conducting genomics have been developed. The Sanger method involves random fragmentation of single-stranded DNA samples, and replication using polymerase chain reaction. This involves combining samples with labeled dideoxynucleotide bases, primer, polymerase, and DNA bases. Replication of DNA

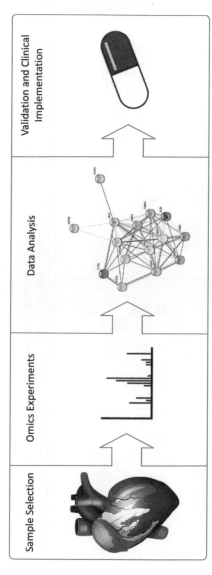

Fig. 1. Process of HF biomarker discovery. In discovering HF biomarkers, first the sample must be acquired. This can be either directly acquired cardiac tissue for measuring local markers, or blood sera or urine to measure circulating markers. The sample then undergoes genomics, transcriptomics, proteomics, or metabolomics either in isolation or using a combination of methods. Data are analyzed using artificial intelligence methods such as principal components analysis, random forest, and support vector machine models. After marker discovery, results can be validated with potential clinical utility as prognostic or diagnostic markers and druggable targets.

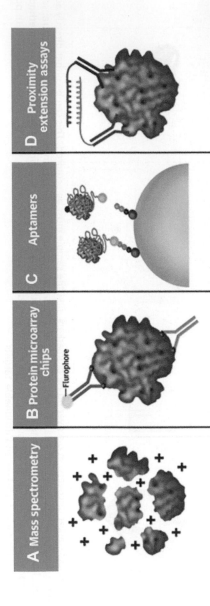

Fig. 2. Proteomic methods. Proteomic methods include mass spectrometry (A), protein microarray chips (B), aptamers (C), and proximity extension assays (D). Each method has its strengths and shortcomings, allowing for different utilities depending on the application. (*From* Michelhaugh SA, Januzzi JL. Finding a Needle in a Haystack: Proteomics in Heart Failure. *JACC Basic to Transl Sci.* 2020;5(10):1043-1053; with permission.)

strands will occur until random inclusion of a dideoxynucleotide base. The samples are then separated by size using gel electrophoresis and labeled dideoxynucleotide give information regarding terminal base and distance traveled gives size. Combining this information with the other fragments provides the DNA sequence.[25,29–31] Today other platforms such as DNA microarrays (discussed in the proteomics section) are used as they are higher throughput for identifying single nucleotide polymorphisms and are less prone to experimental error.[29,31]

Transcriptomics

Transcriptomics studies the ribonucleic acid (RNA) expressed by a cell both involved in coding proteins (mRNA, rRNA, and tRNA) and noncoding RNA (**Fig. 3**). Coding RNA gives insights into the proteins translated by the cell and noncoding shows possible posttranscriptional modulation of protein translation.[12,20] Other noncoding RNA, notably microRNA (RNA sequences between 18 and 25 nucleotides long) and long noncoding RNA (lncRNA, RNA sequences over 200 nucleotides long) are gaining interest as their role in regulating protein translation is being better understood.[20,32] Characterization of the dynamic transcriptome gives researchers upstream and downstream insight into HF pathologies such as identifying dysregulated genes in HF with preserved ejection fraction (HFpEF).[33] Given the similarity between DNA and RNA, modalities to sequence the genome can be applied to transcriptomics as well. This includes RNA-specific forms of microarrays and Sanger sequencing.[31,34]

Proteomics

Characterization of proteome provides insights into disease states and underlying pathophysiologies at the level of proteins (see **Fig. 3**). Beyond identifying potential biomarkers, proteomics can quantify proteins, determine regulation relative to normal or

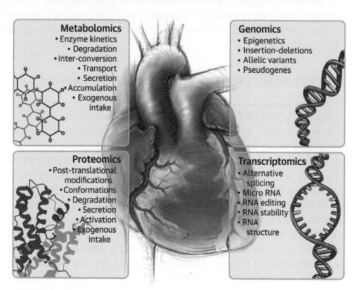

Fig. 3. Overview of omics fields and uses. Omics allows for characterization of the pathophysiology of heart failure in multiple dimensions. As heart failure is a multifaceted disease, a deeper understanding at the level of genes, transcripts, proteins, and metabolites is necessary. (*From* Michelhaugh SA, Januzzi JL. Finding a Needle in a Haystack: Proteomics in Heart Failure. *JACC Basic to Transl Sci.* 2020;5(10):1043-1053; with permission.)

other timepoints, and determine posttranslational modifications such as phosphorylation.[35] Through AI, protein-protein interaction can be determined to elucidate pathophysiology and develop targeted therapies.[12,13,24,36]

Although protein biomarker discovery previously involved hypothesis generation and individual marker testing, modern methods are high throughput with improved sensitivity and selectivity to detect low abundance proteins, and consume minimal sample.[19] The 4 most common modalities of proteomics are mass spectrometry (MS), protein microarrays, aptamer, and proximity extension assays (PEAs), which will be discussed in more detail in the *Approaches* section. These proteomic strategies improve knowledge of HF pathophysiology and can identify potential biomarkers of developing HF, HF diagnostic and prognostic biomarkers, and markers associated with HF prevention, and ultimately improve HF patient care.[8–11]

Metabolomics

The final major omics field is metabolomics, which studies the downstream, metabolic products of cellular processes (see **Fig. 3**). These include amino acids, carbohydrates, fatty acids, nucleic acids, and inorganic molecules.[12,13] In HF research, metabolomics can aid clinicians and researchers in understanding how certain pathologies use different metabolic processes.[37,38] For example, metabolic markers such as phosphatidylcholine and lysophosphatidylcholine (phospholipid metabolites), ornithine (an amino acid metabolite), isocitrate and hydroxybutyrate (cellular energy metabolites), and cotinine (a nicotine metabolite) were associated with an increased risk of developing HF in previously healthy individuals.[38]

Similar to proteomics, MS can characterize the metabolome in an unbiased manner.[12,13] In addition, nuclear magnetic resonance spectroscopy can determine structures, and therein identities of analytes of separated samples using magnetic fields.[12,13,39,40] Likewise, Fourier Transformed Infrared Spectroscopy (FTIR) can identify unknown metabolites, although with less utility as FTIR can only provide information regarding functional groups. However, FTIR is nondestructive and can analyze solid, liquid, or gas samples.[39]

APPROACHES IN PROTEOMICS FOR IDENTIFICATION OF BIOMARKERS
MS Proteomics

MS is a powerful analytical technique for identifying unknown samples. Unlike other proteomic techniques, MS is destructive, as analyte is fragmented before being ionized and sorted by mass-to-charge (m/z) ratio.[41] Using existing libraries, fragments can be pieced together to identify analytes. A benefit of MS is it is untargeted and proteins across the characterized proteome can be detected as well as posttranslational modifications. Despite these advantages, MS may not be as sensitive as other proteomic methods and has limited ability to detect low-abundance proteins.

Standard methods for MS include sample separation using liquid chromatography (LC) or 2-dimensional gel electrophoresis (2-DE). The basis of LC separation is the relative affinity of an analyte for the mobile or stationary phase will cause the various proteins to elute from the column at different times allowing for separation; resolution can be improved by changing the polarity of the different phases.[41,42] In 2-DE, an unknown protein mixture is separated on a gel matrix first by pH until the protein reaches its isoelectric point (has no net charge), and then perpendicularly using electrophoresis to separate proteins by mass.[43,44] Although both methods can be fine-tuned to improve separation, LC is more common as it produces better resolution and is easily coupled to MS instruments.

After separation, samples must be ionized, usually using either matrix-assisted laser desorption ionization or electrospray ionization.[41,45] After ionization, the fragments must be separated by m/z ratio using either time of flight (TOF) or quadrupole analyzers. The m/z ratios of fragments findings can be compared to databases such as the National Institute of Standards and Technology.[46] Although identification of peptides from fragments was once a tedious process, machine learning has increased the ease of this process by generating algorithms to optimize identification processes.[47]

Protein Microarray Proteomics

Microarrays permit the analysis of numerous unknown analytes simultaneously.[48,49] Besides being used in proteomics, microarrays have applications in genomics and transcriptomics.[31] Microarrays can identify, quantify, and determine protein interactions, but are limited as they are relatively targeted by nature, limited to established antibody libraries, and do not have a high binding affinity with target proteins compared with other platforms.[48,49] In proteomics, 2 main modalities of microarrays are used: analytical and functional microarrays.

Analytical microarrays aim to identify and quantify proteins that are differentially regulated. Although there are several methods, the most common involves capture antibodies which have previously been determined to have binding affinity for target proteins are attached to a plate. Next, the sample is added to the plate and binding occurs if the antibody is specific for the protein. A reporter antibody with fluorescent or radioactive marker is then added and attaches to the capture antibody-protein complex. The complex can then be detected and quantified to provide information about the sample.[50] In functional microarrays, the identified proteins of interest are attached to the plate and are exposed to conditions such as drugs, lipids, DNA, and RNA to determine protein interactions.[49]

Aptamer Proteomics

Much like microarray proteomics, aptamer proteomics allows for testing numerous proteins simultaneously based on binding affinity to a previously characterized target. However, in this proteomics modality, short, tightly coiled oligonucleotide strands rather than antibodies are used. This difference creates more specific binding of aptamer to protein compared with protein microarrays.[51] Higher specificity is the result of aptamer design, and the complex sample processing, which has multiple steps to remove excess reagents and off-target binding products.[16,51,52]

Despite these successes, aptamer proteomics has its shortcomings. First, as it is relatively targeted because of the limited aptamer library, it has the potential of introducing bias in the analysis. The results generated from aptamer proteomics are relative concentrations, which cannot be compared to findings from other assays.[52] The sample processing involves multiple steps, introducing the possibility of human error.[51] The specificity of aptamer to protein introduces possible concerns. Although there is strong specificity for aptamers for target proteins, there is potential for cross-reactivity of different protein targets if the sequence and structure are conserved at the aptamer binding site.[10] The high affinity binding may not occur if there are posttranslational modifications.

PEA Proteomics

PEA is a proteomics method with great promise in biomarker discovery. Like microarrays, PEA involves binding of 2 antibodies to proteins in the sample. Instead of using radioactive or fluorescent markers, the protein-binding antibodies contain complimentary, short, single-stranded oligonucleotide sequences on the F_c region. The antibodies are designed so the F_{ab} portions bind the target protein in proximity such that the oligonucleotides will hybridize. The hybridized oligonucleotide can be amplified using quantitative polymerase chain reaction.[53,54]

Advantages of PEA over other proteomics platforms is high sensitivity, reduced cross-reactivity, and ability to detect low concentrations of proteins. PEA only requires 1 µL of sample, making it beneficial when conserving sample for other analyses.[19] Limitations of PEA are inability to detect posttranslational modifications, bias introduced by targeted approach, and currently limited library.[55,56]

STATISTICAL ANALYSIS OF OMICS DATA

In the past, large and complicated data sets generated by omics required extensive statistical analysis. However, increased access to AI has improved analysis of omics data sets. Although there are several methods to analyze omics, the major methods include principal components analysis (PCA), random forest models, and support vector machines (SVMs) (**Table 1**).

PCA allows for related groups of proteins, referred to as features, to be extracted using orthogonal (90°) or oblique (<90°) rotations. Orthogonal rotations have been widely used in HF proteomic research because of the relative ease of analysis. However, this does not depict the one-to-many relationships proteins have in biological systems.[57] Once feature extraction is complete, individual proteins of interest are identified using matrixes.[58]

Random forest models use a series of decision trees to classify data based on supervised teaching data. To construct the random forest, numerous decision trees are created using different variables as the initial nodes and selecting a random number of variables at each step of the tree. From there, a bootstrap aggregate data set is used with the different trees and categorized. Using a system of majority voting where the greatest number of categorizations for one data point, the final classification is determined.[59,60]

SVMs are another form of supervised machine learning used in biomarker discovery analysis. Using training data sets of known classifications, groups are separated using a hyperplane (a line if there are 2 input features and a plane if there are 3 input features). Although many hyperplanes may correctly separate the data, the hyperplane that results in the greatest distance from the points in each cluster closest to the

Table 1
Comparison of omics analysis methods

Method	Strengths	Weaknesses
Principal components analysis	• Reduces overfitting • Reduces noise in data	• Use of oblique rotations is computationally more difficult • Unsupervised learning
Random forest model	• Reduces overfitting • Supervised learning	• Computationally complex • Training period is longer than other methods
Support vector machine	• Supervised learning • Not influenced by outliers	• Prone to overfitting • Does not explain data as well as other methods • Not as effective when datapoints overlap

hyperplane, known as the margin, is chosen. Large margins will aid with classification of data that may otherwise not be as discernible with smaller margins; however, this process may result in overfitting.[8,61]

The function, structure, and interactions of proteins identified can be better understood using AI and established databases. Gene ontology terms define proteins' functions to aid understanding pathophysiology of identified markers. Likewise, the Kyoto Encyclopedia of Genes and Genome provides pathway analysis to shed light on the role of identified proteins in disease mechanisms.[58] Other tools such as the Search Tool for the Retrieval of Interacting Genes/Proteins demonstrates protein-protein interactions.[62] Motif analysis can help gain insight to protein sequence, structure, and posttranslational modifications that may be associated with specific pathologies.[58]

AI has made *in silico* biomarker prediction possible. Although it is not currently used extensively in HF research, other fields have used data sets from several large proteomic studies to generate panels of proteins associated with various cancers[63] and Alzheimer's disease.[64] In hepatocellular carcinoma research, neural networks, a subdivision of machine learning, was used to identify prognostic markers.[65] Although predicted markers will require further validation, AI can economically identify potential biomarkers and conserves samples for biomarker validation.

METHODOLOGIC CONSIDERATIONS

When designing biomarker discovery experiments, there are several considerations. One decision is sample source. Although most proteomics studies test serum, it may be difficult to detect proteins with low expression.[16,52] Other sample types, such as tissue, provide insights to the local proteome within the heart but are difficult to obtain.[66] Urine samples, although easily obtained are not without their shortcomings. Proteins in urine and are more representative of immediate processes and thus is more susceptible to minute-to-minute changes. The urine proteome requires characterization before becoming readily used.[67–69]

After determining sample type, the proteomics modality must be decided. Important considerations include choosing between an untargeted method such as MS (which is better suited for broad marker discovery) or targeted methods such as PEA (which as better suited for validation of previous findings and quantification).[13,70] Some techniques are better suited for certain applications, like using MS if there are concerns of posttranslational modifications affecting binding to aptamers.[71] Proteins involved in specific pathologies may have cross-reactivity, affecting results.[10] Even within a method, other parameters should be adjusted, including separation techniques in MS, and selection of protein panels in PEA, for example.

The final considerations are related to analysis of omics data. When deciding whether to use a targeted versus untargeted approach, targeted methods inherently introduce selection bias.[13,14,17,70,72] Other statistical alterations, such as changing false discovery rates and significance thresholds, for example, have the potential to greatly change data interpretation and results.[57,72] Care must be taken to ensure considerations align with the aims of the interpretation.

EXAMPLES OF STUDIES

The application of proteomics in HF research has uncovered new insights into disease processes. The following studies demonstrate how proteomics of various platforms can be used to discover biomarkers to aid in identifying those at risk for developing HF, predicting disease progression, and understanding mechanism of disease progression and treatments.

MS Proteomics of Urine Samples

Although many studies have applied MS proteomics to discover biomarkers associated with HF with reduced ejection fraction (HFrEF) using blood samples, Rossing and colleagues used urine samples from 127 patients with HFrEF, 581 controls without HF, and 176 with left ventricular diastolic dysfunction (LVDD) to discover potential markers of HFrEF and LVDD.[8] In their experimental design, spontaneous urine samples underwent capillary electrophoresis separation coupled MS using electrospray ionization and TOF analyzer.[8]

In an initial discovery phase, Rossing and colleagues analyzed the proteome of 33 HFrEF patients and 29 age-matched and sex-matched control patients without HF, ultimately identifying 103 peptides associated with HF. These peptides were predominately associated with the extracellular matrix (collagen type I and III and alpha-1-antitrypsin). After identifying peptides, machine learning was used to develop a system of weighting the amplitudes of MS peaks; the model generated was applied to 94 additional HFrEF patients to validate with 93.6% sensitivity, 92.9% specificity, and an area under the curve (AUC) of 0.972 (0.957–0.984, $P < .0001$). Interestingly, among 20 patients with preclinical HFrEF, the model had a sensitivity of 95%.[8]

Protein Microarray Proteomics to Discover Diagnostic and Prognostic Markers

Although not as commonly used as other modalities of proteomics and biomarker discovery, protein microarrays can successfully detect low quantities of proteins.[9] Jiang and colleagues used this platform to gain further insights into HFpEF. Currently, there are fewer markers for diagnosis and prognosis of HFpEF, which negatively impacts care for this patient population. In a small pilot sample of 3 HFpEF patients (defined as having New York Heart Association [NYHA] class III or IV HF, a left ventricular ejection fraction [LVEF] of greater than 40%, and N-terminal B-type natriuretic peptide [NT-proBNP] greater than 1500 pg/mL), 3 hypertensive patients, and 3 healthy control patients, sera samples underwent microarray testing. In their analysis, 507 proteins were tested and ultimately identified 59 significantly upregulated proteins, 11 of which were expressed more than 5-fold greater in HFpEF patients relative to control; 17 proteins were significantly upregulated in HFpEF relative to the hypertensive group and 1 was upregulated 5 times greater. Common to both analyses of being upregulated greater than 5 times to its comparison group was angiogenin.[9]

Angiogenin is a marker of angiogenesis and has previously been thought to be involved in HF pathophysiology.[9,73] After identification of this potential HFpEF biomarker, Jiang and colleagues performed angiogenin immunohistochemistry validation in 16 HFpEF patients (LVEF = 41-49%, n = 9; LVEF $\geq$ 50%, n = 7) and 16 healthy controls. After adjusting for risk factors including age, sex, hypertension, and diabetes, angiogenin was elevated in both HFpEF groups relative to control. However, there was no statistical difference between the 2 ejection fraction cutoffs. When angiogenin was used as a predictor of HFpEF, it was found that the AUC was 0.88 (95% confidence interval, 0.73–1.00; $P < .001$), with a sensitivity of 81% and specificity of 94%. Despite the diagnostic and prognostic power of angiogenin, it did not serve as a predictor of all-cause death at 36-month follow-up.[9]

Aptamer Proteomics to Predict Incident Heart Failure

Prediction of HF using biomarkers is beneficial to clinicians as it allows for more aggressive and targeted interventions to prevent progression. Although markers like NT-proBNP have previously been identified as having predictive value for developing HF, additional markers are needed to better predict progression.[74] Nayor and colleagues aimed to identify protein biomarkers associated with cardiac remodeling as evidenced through echocardiographic parameters using aptamer-based proteomics. In their setup, the investigators included 1895 patients from the Framingham Heart Study without HF at baseline and measured up to 1305 proteins. Protein levels were then compared to various echocardiographic measures; it was ultimately found that 17 proteins were differentially regulated with regards to echocardiographic measures of left ventricular (LV) mass, LV diastolic dimension, and left atrial diameter.[10]

In another prospective analysis, the proteome of 174 patients who developed incident HF from baseline was compared to 1711 individuals who remained HF-free. From this examination, 29 proteins were associated with incident HF. When comparing these 29 potential biomarkers, no statistical difference was observed between those who developed HFpEF and HFrEF. When repeated using samples from the Nord-Trøndelag Health Study (n = 2497), a meta-analysis of the 149 patients with incident HF and 174 from the Framingham Heart Study yielded 6 differentially regulated proteins. Three of these proteins were upregulated (NT-proBNP, thrombospondin-2, and mannose-binding lectin) and 3 were downregulated (epidermal growth factor receptor, growth differentiation factor 8/11, and hemojuvelin).[10]

Nayor and colleagues identified proteins associated with HF development measured with a mean of 19 years before follow-up in the Framingham Heart Study cohort. This suggests possible prediction of incident HF and identification of at-risk patients after further validation.

PEA to Identify Potential Targets to Prevent or Treat Heart Failure

Identifying specific interventions to prevent the development of HF remains a goal of HF clinicians. Although some treatments prevent progression to HF, notably β-blockers, angiotensin receptor blockers, and angiotensin-converting enzyme inhibitors, gaining a better mechanistic understanding of how these therapies prevent HF development will allow for more targeted therapeutic interventions in the future.[11,75] Using PEA proteomics, Ferreira and colleagues hoped to describe the mechanism of how spironolactone, a mineralocorticoid receptor antagonist, is able to improve survival in HF patients and prevent HF development.

In a randomized trial of adults aged 65 years or older receiving spironolactone (n = 265) or standard of care (n = 262), targeted PEA was performed on samples collected from baseline and follow-up at 1 and 9 months after enrollment to measure 276 proteins. Relative to control, those receiving spironolactone significantly downregulated 18 proteins and upregulated 33 proteins between baseline and 9 months after enrollment. When also examining changes between baseline, 1-, and 9-month follow-up samples, 5 proteins were significantly downregulated and 14 were significantly upregulated. Using network analysis, the 10 most differentially regulated proteins were assigned to 3 different clusters of 6 biologic functions (adipocytokine signaling, renin-angiotensin-aldosterone pathway, extracellular matrix metabolism, insulin growth factor signaling, hemostasis, and immune response).[11]

These different functional groupings reflect the possible effect of spironolactone on remodeling processes involved in HF such as decreasing collagen synthesis, inflammation, and angiogenesis. Better characterization and directed therapeutic interventions may prevent progression of patients at risk from developing HF.[11]

In another study, PEA was used to evaluate changes in the proteome of individuals with HFrEF before and after initiation of angiotensin receptor/neprilysin inhibitor (ARNI) in those with moderately advanced HF and following unloading with left ventricular assist device (LVAD) placement among those with advanced HF. In this analysis, Michelhaugh and colleagues found 5 proteins (NT-proBNP, endothelial cell-specific molecule-1, cathepsin L1, osteopontin, and MCSF-1) were differentially regulated after treatment with ARNI and LVAD. This core protein signature for HF may serve as a more accurate diagnostic cluster for the diagnosis, serve as druggable targets, have prognostic utility, or be used to monitor HF care.[76]

SUMMARY

Advancements in omics and AI have improved researcher's ability to discover HF biomarkers. Rather than relying on hypothesis-driven, individual marker testing, omics has opened the door to high-throughput analyses of genome, transcriptome, proteome, and metabolome to gain deeper understandings of pathophysiology in HF. With future validation studies, the characterized markers can be developed into panels to predict and monitor HF in the clinic. Discovered markers can be used as targets to treat HF patients or design therapeutic interventions to prevent HF from developing in at-risk patients. As AI and omics technologies continue to evolve, the clinical utility will increase substantially, improving patient outcomes.

CLINICS CARE POINTS

- Greater accessibility to AI allows clinical researchers to expand biomarker prediction and discovery.
- Although powerful at discovering potential markers, further validation is required before implementing at the bedside.
- AI can potentially predict biomarkers associated with HF using previously measured omics data.
- Integration of multiple biomarkers increases understanding of heart failure pathophysiology, and clinically can aid in improving detection, treatments, and quality of life.

DISCLOSURE

Dr J.L. Januzzi is supported in part by the Hutter Family Professorship; has been a trustee of the American College of Cardiology; has received grant support from Novartis Pharmaceuticals and Abbott Diagnostics; has received consulting income from Abbott, Janssen, Novartis, and Roche Diagnostics; has participated in clinical endpoint committees/data safety monitoring boards for Abbott, AbbVie, Amgen, CVRx, Janssen, MyoKardia, and Takeda. Mr S.A. Michelhaugh has no relationships to disclose.

REFERENCES

1. Yancy CW, Jessup M, Chair V, et al. Practice Guideline 2013 ACCF/AHA Guideline for the Management of Heart Failure. J Am Coll Cardiol. 2013 Oct 15;62(16):e147–239.
2. Troughton RW, Frampton CM, Yandle TG, et al. Treatment of heart failure guided by plasma aminoterminal brain natriuretic peptide (N-BNP) concentrations. Lancet 2000;355(9210):1126–30.
3. Troughton R, Felker GM, Januzzi JL. Natriuretic peptide-guided heart failure management. doi:10.1093/eurheartj/eht463

4. Giannessi D. Multimarker approach for heart failure management: Perspectives and limitations. Pharma Res 2011;64(1):11–24.

5. Pemberton CJ, Ikeda Y, De Rosa S, et al. The Diagnostic and Therapeutic Value of Multimarker Analysis in Heart Failure. An Approach to Biomarker-Targeted Therapy. Front Cardiovasc Med 2020;7:579567. www.frontiersin.org.

6. Burchfield JS, Xie M, Hill JA. Pathological ventricular remodeling: Mechanisms: Part 1 of 2. Circulation 2013;128(4):388–400.

7. Holzhauser L, Kim G, Sayer G, et al. The Effect of Left Ventricular Assist Device Therapy on Cardiac Biomarkers: Implications for the Identification of Myocardial Recovery. Curr Heart Fail Rep. 2018 Aug;15(4):250–259.

8. Rossing K, Bosselmann HS, Gustafsson F, et al. Urinary proteomics pilot study for biomarker discovery and diagnosis in heart failure with reduced ejection fraction. PLoS One 2016;11(6):e0157167.

9. Jiang H, Zhang L, Yu Y, et al. A pilot study of angiogenin in heart failure with preserved ejection fraction: a novel potential biomarker for diagnosis and prognosis? J Cell Mol Med. 2014 Nov;18(11):2189–97.

10. Nayor M, Short MI, Rasheed H, et al. Aptamer-Based Proteomic Platform Identifies Novel Protein Predictors of Incident Heart Failure and Echocardiographic Traits. Circ Hear Fail 2020;13(5). https://doi.org/10.1161/CIRCHEARTFAILURE. 119.006749.

11. Ferreira JP, Verdonschot J, Wang P, et al. Proteomic and Mechanistic Analysis of Spironolactone in Patients at Risk for HF. JACC Hear Fail 2021;9(4):268–77.

12. Hasin Y, Seldin M, Lusis A. Multi-omics approaches to disease. Genome Biol. 2017 May 5;18(1):8.

13. Vailati-Riboni M, Palombo V, Loor JJ. What are omics sciences?. In: Periparturient diseases of Dairy Cows: a systems Biology approach. Springer International Publishing; 2017. p. 1–7. https://doi.org/10.1007/978-3-319-43033-1_1.

14. Subramanian I, Verma S, Kumar S, et al. Multi-omics Data Integration, Interpretation, and Its Application. Bioinform Biol Insights 2020;14. https://doi.org/10.1177/1177932219899051.

15. Ahmad T, Fiuzat M, Pencina MJ, et al. Charting a Roadmap for Heart Failure Biomarker Studies NIH Public Access. JACC Hear Fail 2014;2(5):477–88.

16. Brody EN, Gold L, Lawn RM, et al. High-content affinity-based proteomics: Unlocking protein biomarker discovery. Expert Rev Mol Diagn 2010;10(8):1013–22.

17. Zheng Y. Study Design Considerations for Cancer Biomarker Discoveries. J Appl Lab Med 2018;3(2):282–9.

18. McDermott JE, Wang J, Mitchell H, et al. Challenges in biomarker discovery: Combining expert insights with statistical analysis of complex omics data. Expert Opin Med Diagn 2013;7(1):37–51.

19. Smith JG, Gerszten RE. Emerging affinity-based proteomic technologies for large-scale plasma profiling in cardiovascular disease. Circulation 2017; 135(17):1651–64.

20. Chambers DC, Carew AM, Lukowski SW, et al. Transcriptomics and single-cell RNA-sequencing. Respirology 2019;24(1):29–36.

21. Kulkarni A, Anderson AG, Merullo DP, et al. Beyond bulk: A review of single cell transcriptomics methodologies and applications Graphical abstract HHS Public Access Author manuscript. Curr Opin Biotechnol 2019;58:129–36.

22. Lancellotti C, Cancian P, Savevski V, et al. Artificial Intelligence & Tissue Biomarkers: Advantages, Risks and Perspectives for Pathology. 2021. Cells. 2021 Apr 2;10(4):787.

23. D'adamo GL, Widdop JT, Giles EM, et al. The future is now? Clinical and translational aspects of "Omics" technologies. Immunol Cell Biol 2021;99:168–76.
24. Chen C, Hou J, Tanner JJ, et al. Molecular Sciences Bioinformatics Methods for Mass Spectrometry-Based Proteomics Data Analysis. Int J Mol Sci. 2020 Apr 20;21(8):2873.
25. Del Giacco L, Cattaneo C. Introduction to genomics. Methods Mol Biol 2012;823:79–88.
26. Smith NL, Felix JF, Morrison AC, et al. Association of genome-wide variation with the risk of incident heart failure in adults of European and African ancestry : A prospective meta-analysis from the cohorts for heart and aging research in genomic epidemiology (CHARGE) consortium. Circ Cardiovasc Genet 2010; 3(3):256–66.
27. Reza N, Owens AT. Advances in the Genetics and Genomics of Heart Failure. Curr Cardiol Rep 2020;22(11). https://doi.org/10.1007/s11886-020-01385-z.
28. Tayal U, Prasad S, Cook SA. Genetics and genomics of dilated cardiomyopathy and systolic heart failure. Genome Med 2017;9(1). https://doi.org/10.1186/s13073-017-0410-8.
29. Wright J. A primer on DNA sequencing for the practicing urologist. Urol Times Urol Cancer Care 2021;10(2). Available at: https://www.urologytimes.com/view/a-primer-on-dna-sequencing-for-the-practicing-urologist.
30. Shendure J, Balasubramanian S, Church GM, et al. DNA sequencing at 40: Past, present and future. Nature 2017;550(7676):345–53.
31. Gasperskaja E, Kučinskas V. The most common technologies and tools for functional genome analysis. Acta Med Litu 2017;24(1):1–11.
32. Fang Y, Fullwood MJ. Roles, Functions, and Mechanisms of Long Non-coding RNAs in Cancer. Genomics Proteomics Bioinformatics 2016;14(1):42–54.
33. Das S, Frisk C, Eriksson MJ, et al. Transcriptomics of cardiac biopsies reveals differences in patients with or without diagnostic parameters for heart failure with preserved ejection fraction. Sci Rep. 2019 Feb 28;9(1):3179.
34. Valdés A, Ibáñez C, Simó C, et al. Recent transcriptomics advances and emerging applications in food science. Trac - Trends Anal Chem 2013;52:142–54.
35. Mann M, Jensen ON. Proteomic analysis of post-translational modifications. Nat Biotechnol 2003;21(3):255–61.
36. Michelhaugh SA, Januzzi JL. Finding a Needle in a Haystack: Proteomics in Heart Failure. JACC Basic Transl Sci 2020;5(10):1043–53.
37. Tahir UA, Katz DH, Zhao T, et al. Metabolomic profiles and heart failure risk in black adults: Insights from the jackson heart study. Circ Heart Fail. 2021 Jan;14(1):e007275.
38. Andersson C, Liu C, Cheng S, et al. Metabolomic signatures of cardiac remodelling and heart failure risk in the community. ESC Hear Fail 2020;7(6):3707–15.
39. Bujak R, Struck-Lewicka W, Markuszewski MJ, et al. Metabolomics for laboratory diagnostics. J Pharm Biomed Anal 2015;113:108–20.
40. Kordalewska M, Markuszewski MJ. Metabolomics in cardiovascular diseases. J Pharm Biomed Anal 2015;113:121–36.
41. Timp W, Timp G. Beyond mass spectrometry, the next step in proteomics. Sci Adv 2020;6(2):eaax8978.
42. Ali I, Aboul-Enein HY, Singh P, et al. Separation of biological proteins by liquid chromatography. Saudi Pharm J 2010;18(2):59–73.
43. Ning F, Wu X, Wang W. Expert Review of Proteomics Exploiting the potential of 2DE in proteomics analyses Exploiting the potential of 2DE in proteomics analyses. Expert Rev Proteomics. 2016 Oct;13(10):901–3.

44. Lohnes K, Quebbemann NR, Liu K, et al. Combining high-throughput MALDI-TOF mass spectrometry and isoelectric focusing gel electrophoresis for virtual 2D gel-based proteomics. Methods 2016;104:163–9.
45. Aebersold R, Mann M. Mass spectrometry-based proteomics. Nature 2003; 422(6928):198–207.
46. Stein S. Mass spectral reference libraries: An ever-expanding resource for chemical identification. Anal Chem 2012;84(17):7274–82.
47. Liebal UW, Phan ANT, Sudhakar M, et al. Machine learning applications for mass spectrometry-based metabolomics. Metabolites 2020;10(6):1–23.
48. Zhu H, Qian J. Applications of Functional Protein Microarrays in Basic and Clinical Research. Advances in genetics, 79. Academic Press Inc.; 2012. p. 123–55. https://doi.org/10.1016/B978-0-12-394395-8.00004-9.
49. Hu S, Xie Z, Qian J, et al. Functional Protein Microarray Technology. Wiley Interdiscip Rev Syst Biol Med 2011;3(3):255–68.
50. Macbeath G. Protein microarrays and proteomics. Nat Genet 2002;32(4S): 526–32.
51. Gold L, Ayers D, Bertino J, et al. Aptamer-based multiplexed proteomic technology for biomarker discovery. PLoS One 2010;5(12). https://doi.org/10.1371/journal.pone.0015004.
52. Lollo B, Steele F, Gold L. Beyond antibodies: New affinity reagents to unlock the proteome. Proteomics 2014;14(6):638–44.
53. Assarsson E, Lundberg M, Holmquist G, et al. Homogenous 96-plex PEA immunoassay exhibiting high sensitivity, specificity, and excellent scalability. PLoS One 2014;9(4):e95192.
54. Lundberg M, Eriksson A, Tran B, et al. Homogeneous antibody-based proximity extension assays provide sensitive and specific detection of low-abundant proteins in human blood. Nucleic Acids Res. 2011 Aug;39(15):e102.
55. Solier C, Langen H. Antibody-based proteomics and biomarker research-current status and limitations. Proteomics 2014;14(6):774–83.
56. Graumann J, Finkernagel F, Reinartz S, et al. Multi-platform Affinity Proteomics Identify Proteins Linked to Metastasis and Immune Suppression in Ovarian Cancer Plasma. Front Oncol 2019;9:1150.
57. Lualdi M, Fasano M. Statistical analysis of proteomics data: A review on feature selection. J Proteomics 2019;198:18–26.
58. Schmidt A, Forne I, Imhof A. Bioinformatic analysis of proteomics data. BMC Syst Biol 2014;8(Suppl 2):S3.
59. Yang L, Wu H, Jin X, et al. Study of cardiovascular disease prediction model based on random forest in eastern China. Sci Rep 2020;10(1). https://doi.org/10.1038/S41598-020-62133-5.
60. Breiman L. Random Forests. Mach Learn 45, 5–32 (2001).
61. Cortes C. Support-Vector Networks. Mach Learn 20, 273–297 (1995).
62. Szklarczyk D, Gable AL, Lyon D, et al. STRING v11: Protein-protein association networks with increased coverage, supporting functional discovery in genome-wide experimental datasets. Nucleic Acids Res 2019;47(D1):D607–13.
63. Björling E, Lindskog C, Oksvold P, et al. A web-based tool for in silico biomarker discovery based on tissue-specific protein profiles in normal and cancer tissues. Mol Cell Proteomics 2008;7(5):825–44.
64. Greco I, Day N, Riddoch-Contreras J, et al. Alzheimer's disease biomarker discovery using in silico literature mining and clinical validation. J Transl Med 2012;10(1):1–10.

65. Chaudhary K, Poirion OB, Lu L, et al. Deep Learning based multi-omics integration robustly predicts survival in liver cancer. Clin Cancer Res 2018;24(6):1248.

66. Lam MPY, Ping P, Murphy E. Proteomics Research in Cardiovascular Medicine and Biomarker Discovery. J Am Coll Cardiol 2016;68(25):2819–30.

67. Gao YH. Urine-an untapped goldmine for biomarker discovery? Sci China Life Sci 2013;56(12):1145–6.

68. Jing J, Gao Y. Urine Biomarkers in the Early Stages of Diseases: Current Status and Perspective - Jian Jing - Discovery Medicine. Discov Med 2018;25(136):57–65. Available at: https://www.discoverymedicine.com/Jian-Jing-2/2018/02/urine-biomarkers-in-the-early-stages-of-diseases-current-status-and-perspective/.

69. Gao Y. Urine is a better biomarker source than blood especially for kidney diseases. Adv Exp Med Biol 2015;845:3–12.

70. Sobsey CA, Ibrahim S, Richard VR, et al. Targeted and Untargeted Proteomics Approaches in Biomarker Development. Proteomics 2020;20(9). https://doi.org/10.1002/pmic.201900029.

71. Betzen C, Alhamdani MSS, Lueong S, et al. Clinical proteomics: Promises, challenges and limitations of affinity arrays. Proteomics - Clin Appl 2015;9(3–4):342–7.

72. Lay JO, Borgmann S, Liyanage R, et al. Problems with the '"omics. "' Trends Anal Chem 2006;25(11):1046–56.

73. Tello-Montoliu A, Patel JV. Lip GYH. Angiogenin: A review of the pathophysiology and potential clinical applications. J Thromb Haemost 2006;4(9):1864–74.

74. Campbell DJ, Gong FF, Jelinek MV, et al. Prediction of incident heart failure by serum amino-terminal pro-B-type natriuretic peptide level in a community-based cohort. Eur J Heart Fail 2019;21(4):449–59.

75. Horwich TB, Fonarow GC. Prevention of heart failure. JAMA Cardiol 2017;2(1):116.

76. Michelhaugh SA, Camacho A, Ibrahim NE, et al. Proteomic Signatures During Treatment in Different Stages of Heart Failure. Circ Hear Fail 2020. https://doi.org/10.1161/circheartfailure.119.006794.

Laboratory Aspects of Minimal / Measurable Residual Disease Testing in B-Lymphoblastic Leukemia

John Kim Choi, MD, PhD[a],*, Paul E. Mead, PhD, SCYM(ASCP)[b]

KEYWORDS

- Minimal residual disease • MRD • B lymphoblastic leukemia • B-ALL
- Leukemia-associated immunophenotype • LAIP

KEY POINTS

- Minimal residual disease detection provides critical prognostic predictor of treatment outcome and is the standard of care for B lymphoblastic leukemia.
- Flow cytometry–based minimal residual disease detection is the most common test modality and has high sensitivity (0.01%) and rapid turnaround time (24 hours).
- Flow cytometry–based minimal residual disease detection is complicated by variabilities on the antigens examined, combination of antibodies, criteria for the blast numerator, criteria for the cells that defines the denominator, and the approach to flow cytometry data analysis.
- Despite these differences, the final minimal residual disease values show similar clinical outcomes.
- Leukemia-associated immunophenotype analysis is simplified by guide gates that define normal B-cell populations and is more accurate using back-gating to include all B-lymphoblastic leukemia cells and exclude contaminating events.

INTRODUCTION

Detection of minimal residual disease (MRD) is a critical prognostic predictor and has become the standard of care[1] for B-lymphoblastic leukemia (B-ALL) in response to up front chemotherapy and success in bone marrow (BM) transplantation for relapsed and high-risk ALL.[2–6] First shown in the pediatric population, similar usefulness has

This article originally appeared in Clinics in Laboratory Medicine, Volume 41 Issue 3, September 2021.

[a] Division of Laboratory Medicine, The University of Alabama at Birmingham, WP P230N, 619 19th Street South, Birmingham, AL 35249-7331, USA; [b] Department of Pathology, St. Jude Children's Research Hospital, 262 Danny Thomas Place, D4026G, Mailstop 342, Memphis, TN 38105, USA

* Corresponding author.

E-mail address: johnchoi@uabmc.edu

https://doi.org/10.1016/j.cll.2022.09.022
0272-2712/23/© 2022 Elsevier Inc. All rights reserved.

labmed.theclinics.com

been shown for the adult population.[7–9] Over time and with the introduction of even more sensitive assays, the threshold for minimal is changing and MRD is being redefined as measurable residual disease.

MRD is often defined as disease below the level of reliable detection by morphology or 5% blasts of the total marrow cellularity.[10] Flow cytometry studies have shown that this 5% value is not very sensitive and values as low at 0.01% residual disease during treatment are predictive of relapse.[2–5] In addition, high percentages (>5%) of normal precursor B cells or lymphoblasts can be seen in normal or regenerating marrow without residual leukemia,[11–13] and can complicate disease status determination when using morphology alone or even standard immunophenotyping by flow cytometry. Currently, there is no consensus for the exact MRD percentage for relapse after patient achieve negative MRD. Some institutions use 1% to define relapse, but others such as St. Jude Children's Research Hospital (SJCRH) still use 5%.

CLINICAL MINIMAL RESIDUAL DISEASE TESTING

Currently, flow cytometry is the most common test modality for MRD with a reliable sensitivity of 0.01% and this percentage is used as the threshold for MRD positivity in most clinical treatment strategies. Other modalities with equal to or greater sensitivity include allelic specific quantitative polymerase chain reaction (PCR), using a primer specific for patient leukemic T-cell receptor or B-cell receptor (IgH or IgL) rearrangement[14] or quantitative reverse transcriptase PCR for fusion transcripts in some leukemia with recurrent chromosomal rearrangement,[15,16] both with a sensitivity of 0.001%. More recent approaches have even higher level of sensitivity of 0.0001%. These approaches include next-generation sequencing (NGS) using linear PCR amplification of T-cell receptor or B-cell receptor rearrangements followed by sequencing and comparing the products to the signature leukemic sequences identified at diagnosis.[17] This approach has a sensitivity of 1 cell in 1 million or 0.0001% and, in certain circumstances, residual disease at even less than 0.01% is predictive of outcome.[18,19] Digital droplet PCR, the latest version of quantitative PCR, is being evaluated in small studies with similar sensitivity to NGS.[20,21]

Two studies have examined the clinical significance of MRD detected by flow cytometry compared with allelic-specific quantitative PCR[22] or with NGS.[19] PCR, as expected with its better sensitivity, can detect residual disease in some of the flow MRD negative cases, but missed some detected by flow, possibly because of clonal evolution and sequence drift. NGS using 0.01% positivity cutoff detected all flow positive cases and identified additional cases that were negative by flow. Outcomes for these 2 studies were similar, relapse occurred most frequently when MRD is positive with both test modalities and least frequently when negative for both tests. In patients where the MRD was positive on only 1 testing platform (either flow- or nucleic acid-based MRD methodologies) an intermediate level of relapse (event-free survival) was observed compared with high- or standard-risk patients.

The remainder of this article focuses on the flow cytometry–based MRD detection for B-ALL that is used by many institutions. This modality is the most common method and has advantages of rapid turnaround time (MRD results reported usually within one working day compared with 7–10 days for the other modalities) and its availability in most clinical laboratories. There is no consensus on the timing, preparation, acquisition, and analysis of flow cytometry. Despite all the variability in flow-based assays, MRD findings in multiple published large studies are equivalent with similar levels of sensitivity and correlation to outcome.[2,5,23–25]

Timing for Flow Cytometry Analysis

Flow-based MRD assays are done on peripheral blood or BM aspirate, typically anti-coagulated with EDTA or heparin and assayed within 24 hours; but can be assayed as late 72 hours if heparin is used as an anticoagulant. The Children's Oncology Group (COG) typically performed MRD analysis on day 8 peripheral blood and 29 BM of chemotherapy,[2] time points with fewer complicating normal precursor B cells. In contrast, MRD studies for the EuroFlow consortium are done at days 15, 33, and 78,[26,27] whereas for SJCRH, MRD studies are done on day 8 peripheral blood and at every BM aspiration (ie, days 15, 21/22 [if MRD >0.1% at day 15], 43, 49, 119, 296, and 840).[5] MRD at both early and later time points are prognostic indicators.[2,5,28]

Preparation and Acquisition of Sample

Currently, COG, EuroFlow, and SJCRH use a lyse approach to remove the non-nucleated red blood cells, but before 2019 SJCRH used Ficoll gradient to remove the red blood cells. Multiple tubes, each containing 0.5 to 4.0 million cells each are stained with 6 to 10 different antibodies to eventually quantify the residual leukemic cells of interest. A wide variety of different antibodies in different combinations are used by different institutions (see **Table 1** for examples) to distinguish the leukemic cells. In addition to the tubes containing fluorescent molecule conjugated antibodies, COG and SJCRH also have another tube with a nuclear stain (Syto 16 or 13, respectively) to help define the denominator (all nucleated cells). In contrast, EuroFlow and French Consortium use only FSC/SSC exclusion to exclude debris and assume that lysis, or Ficoll separation, has removed all non-nucleated red blood cells.

After staining, a total of 0.5 to 1.0 million, 4.0 million, and all stained cells are acquired on the flow cytometry machine by COG, EuroFlow, and SJCRH, respectively. The large number of total events are collected to reach the sensitivity of 0.01% MRD, a value calculated by the total number of leukemic cells divided by the total number of nucleated cells. The derivation of both the numerator and the denominator varies by institution. In general, the leukemic population is considered real if the population is tightly clustered (a subjective criterion) and is composed of 10 or more events, but other institutions require greater numbers.[29,30] With 10 required leukemic

---

Table 1
Antibodies and analysis approaches used by different groups

Group[ref]	COG[11]	EuroFlow[26]	French[25]	SJCRH[28]
Antibodies used: In all tubes	*CD45, CD19, CD10, CD9, CD13/CD33, CD20, CD34, CD38, CD58*	*CD45, CD19, CD10, CD20, CD34, CD38, CD81, CD66c/CD123, CD73/CD304*	*CD45, CD19, CD10, CD2, CD13, CD15, CD20, CD21, CD22, CD24, CD33, CD34, CD38, CD117, CD123*	*CD45, CD19, CD10, CD34, CD22, CD13, CD15, CD20, CD24, CD33, CD38, CD44, CD58, CD66c, CD72, CD73, CD86, CD123, CD133, CD200, NG2 (7.1)*
Analysis approach	Different from normal	Different from normal	LAIP	LAIP
Reported MRD % of what cells (denominator)	Mononuclear cells	Total cells	Total cells	Nucleated mononuclear cells

Abbreviation: LAIP, leukemia-associated immunophenotype.

events, a total of 100,000 single, viable, nucleated cell events are needed to reach 0.01% sensitivity; if 50 leukemic events are required to form a positive cluster, then 500,000 gated events are required to reach the 0.01% threshold. The denominator number also varies by institution. EuroFlow uses all nucleated cells (SSC/FSC exclusion of debris) as the denominator, whereas COG and SJCRH use nucleated mononuclear cells (using nucleic acid-binding [Syto] dyes and high SSC exclusion) as the denominator because their initial assays were developed using Ficolled specimens. Upon transition to a bulk-lysis approach, COG uses a digital gate to exclude all the granulocytes to get the mononuclear cell number. SJCRH also uses a digital gate but removes only the granulocytes that have higher SSC than monocytes because this number empirically correlates with the Ficolled sample. An obvious implication is that the EuroFlow denominator better correlates with the denominator used in NGS studies compared with that used by COG and SJCRH.

Analysis Approaches (Different from Normal versus the Leukemia-Associated Immunophenotype)

How the leukemic cells are determined also differs between the groups. Both COG and EuroFlow use a different from normal approach. With experience, leukemic cells (if sufficient in number and tightly clustered) differ from normal precursor B cells maturation pattern by their shape and location on scatter plots (**Fig. 1**). This approach results in variabilities in interlaboratory results.[31] The implementation of a quality assurance program has improved the concordance probably secondary to some guidelines and possibly secondary to decreased number of laboratories performing flow-based MRD.[32,33] Among experts, the concordance of the results is much better. EuroFlow reports 98% concordance in flow-based MRD analysis among 4 centers indicating low, but not absent, variability among experts and 98% concordance with NGS studies.[26] The exact methodology for the different from normal approach is beyond the scope of this article, and its introduction can be found in recent reviews.[30,34]

The other analysis approach, the leukemia-associated immunophenotype, used by St. Jude Children's Research Hospital and the French consortium will be detailed

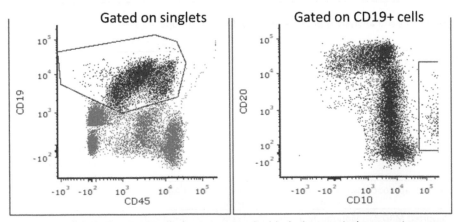

Fig. 1. Normal maturing BM B cells, hematogones (in *blue*), show typical maturation pattern for CD19, CD45, C20, and CD10. Minimal/measurable residual B lymphoblastic leukemia (in *red*) shows aberrant decreased expression of CD45 and increased expression of CD10. Both abnormalities are lost later in treatment.

because of its familiarity to the authors and its easy teachability to others. In the leukemia-associated immunophenotype approach, the leukemic cells are analyzed at diagnosis and a fingerprint of abnormal antigen expression is identified and used to follow the leukemic cells during treatment. In actuality, the leukemia-associated immunophenotype approach is similar to the DNF approach except only the initial abnormality is used as a leukemic marker rather than any abnormality.

SJCRH uses guide gates as an aide for the inexperienced user to distinguish leukemic cells from normal regenerating B-lymphoblasts. Normal regenerating BM (20–25 cases) were used to define the normal pattern of expression for every combination of antibodies used in the B-ALL MRD diagnostic screening panel. A gate was drawn around the normal expression patterns that defines the limits of normal regenerating precursor B cells (frequently referred to as hematogones). Similar normal guide gates have been described by others.[35] Diagnostic marrow is queried with the full panel of potential B-ALL MRD markers, and the best 4 to 6 markers are included for follow-up studies; a Boolean gating scheme is used to define the leukemic population at diagnosis (**Fig. 2**). Although some antigen expressions change during treatment as COG has shown,[36] we find that most abnormal markers remain abnormal. We also find that CD45, CD19, CD10, and CD34 expression are frequently altered in the leukemic cell population, and thus we used these markers as a backbone in each tube of the patient-specific panel and used mainly to identify B cells and their stage of differentiation. The best 4 to 6 antibodies identified at diagnosis, which distinguish leukemic from normal blasts, are used to fill the remaining slots in the follow-up tubes, and this patient-specific panel is run for all subsequent MRD time points. The initial analysis scheme at diagnosis can be modified during treatment to reflect changes in the

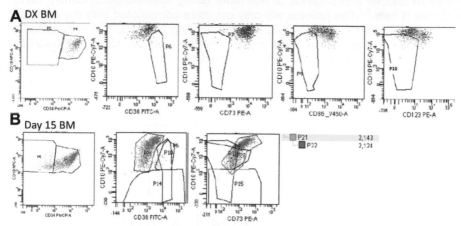

Fig. 2. (*A*) Leukemia-associated immunophenotype (LAIP) is identified at diagnosis. Initial leukemic cells were CD34+, CD10++, and had 4 antigens of varying abnormalities. Gates P4: CD34+CD19+ cells, P5: CD34-CD19+, P6, P7, P9, and P10 represent the boundaries in which hematogones reside for the antigens CD38, CD73, CD86, and CD123, respectively. (*B*) MRD analysis of BM after 15 days of induction shows that the leukemic cells now have variable CD34 and CD10 expression. CD38 decreased further to become a better LAIP marker, whereas CD73 decreased to become a marginal marker. Normal gates for CD34+ and CD34– are superimposed to allow combined analysis of the B-ALL cells and gates P10, 14, P11, P15 represents normal boundaries for the CD34–CD19+ cells. P21 and P22 represent the leukemic cells and Boolean analysis is performed to quantify B-ALL with both abnormalities.

leukemic phenotype in response to treatment. Back-gating is performed on the final leukemic population and is a crucial step to further refine the leukemic gates to include all leukemic blasts and exclude potential noise (**Fig. 3**).

Our approach has the advantage of being simple for new users to learn. Analysis, particularly of regenerating BM at later time points in therapy, can be complicated by the presence of a background of normal precursor B cells (see **Fig. 1**; **Fig. 4**). Our approach is also useful when only 1 population of precursor B cells is observed and the differential includes left-shifted hematogones or leukemic cells (see **Fig. 4**). A disadvantage is that the antibody and instrument setting have to be rigorously controlled to maintain the same level of mean fluorescent intensity on control cells, and ultimately on the leukemic cells; otherwise the guide gates for the normal regenerating B-cell precursors will not be applicable across samples at different time points. This process necessitates retitrating new lots of antibody to give the same mean fluorescent intensity as the previous lot. Another disadvantage is that the normal guide gates are specific to an individual laboratory, must be tediously and manually drawn, and must be determined for any new markers introduced into the diagnostic screening panel. The final disadvantage is that intracellular markers cannot be used as mean fluorescent intensity reproducibility cannot be maintained, at least in our hands.

Minimum Residual Disease of CD19 Negative B-Lymphoblastic Leukemia

B-ALLs are typically distinguished by expression of CD19 and analysis will eventually gate on the CD19-positive population. However, rare B-ALLs have dim to negative CD19 expression. CD19-negative B-ALL is also becoming more frequent with the introduction of anti-CD19 therapy (blinatumomab and CART-19) for high-risk B-ALL. Hence, the analysis must take into account this possibility by either introduction of CD22 as another B-cell marker or use other gating approaches to identify CD19-negative B cells.[37] This process will only get more complicated with the advent of combined anti-CD19 and anti-CD22 therapy, leading to B-ALL that is negative for both markers (**Fig. 5**). In such cases, SJCRH defines CD19–, intracellular CD79a+ as the leukemic population, with trepidation.

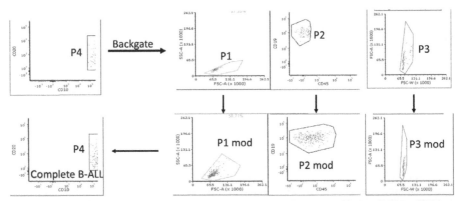

Fig. 3. Back-gate of the initial analysis for B-ALL (P4: CD19+, CD10 bright, CD45 negative). The population in the final leukemic gate is back-gated to all the previous gates. These gates are then modified to include all B-ALL and exclude contaminating cells. In this case, the final population (P4) is back-gated on all the previous gates (P1–3). P1–2 show evidence of exclusion of some B-ALL, whereas P3 shows inclusion of contaminating doublets. P1–3 are modified to include all B-ALL and exclude debris and the new P4 represent all the B-ALL events.

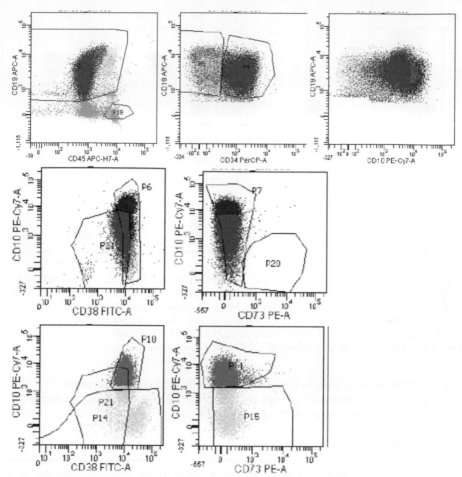

Fig. 4. Left shifted hematogones: Patient with a history of B-ALL, day 43 of treatment. BM with 11% blasts. Analysis shows left shifted hematogones (many at CD34+ and/or CD10+ stage) that lack the aberrant decreased CD38 (P21) or increased CD73 (P20) expression of the B-ALL seen at diagnosis. P6 and 7 represent normal CD34+ B cells. P10, 14, 11, and 15 represent normal CD34- B cells.

Future Advances

More recently, artificial intelligence clustering programs such as tSNE and SPADE have been used to cluster flow data to define and discover normal hematopoietic populations.[38-40] Various laboratories are exploring the possibility of applying these programs to MRD analysis (ie, computer-assisted distinction of leukemic population from normal hematopoietic cells) with promising results.[26,41] These clustering programs are being packaged with current clinical flow cytometry programs, promising that future MRD analysis will become easier and more reproducible.

The current clinical flow cytometry machines are typically limited to 8 to 10 colors. Research-grade flow cytometry can achieve higher numbers,[42] but are impractical in clinical laboratory, mainly owing to technical and regulatory issues. Newer spectral-based flow cytometry instrumentation offers a lot of advantages with many more

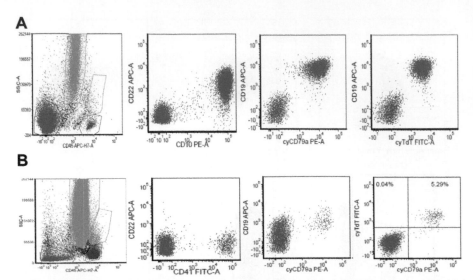

Fig. 5. B-ALL with multiple relapses treated with anti-CD19 and anti-CD22 therapy. (*A*) Initial presentation: B-ALL that is CD45–, CD19+, CD22+, CD10+, CD79a+, and TdT+. (*B*) After anti-CD19 and CD22 therapy. Flow-based MRD is negative, but NGS shows recurrent B-ALL. Peripheral blood immunophenotyping shows abnormal lymphoblasts that are. CD45–, CD19–, CD22–, CD10– (not shown), CD79a+, and TdT+ that was missed on the flow based MRD analysis that gated on CD19+ or CD22+ cells.

colors (>36 markers in a single tube) without need for manual compensation.[43–45] This technology holds promise of a high-parameter single tube analysis, an important benefit when starting with a low cellularity BM sample.

CLINICS CARE POINTS

- Flow based MRD must distinguish residual B lymphoblastic leukemia from normal hematogones.
- In DFN (different from normal) and LAIP (leuekmia associated immunophenotype), the pathologist must have an accurate understanding (often based on years of experience) of normal hematogone flow patterns.
- Analysis can become more objective, and quickly learned by establishing laboratory specific guide gates for normal hematogones.
- Systematic backgating during analysis decreases under and over-estimating MRD.

DISCLOSURE

The authors have no commercial or financial conflicts of interest. This has been funded in part by ALSAC at SJCRH.

REFERENCES

1. Athale UH, Gibson PJ, Bradley NM, et al. Minimal residual disease and childhood leukemia: standard of care recommendations from the Pediatric Oncology Group of Ontario MRD Working Group. Pediatr Blood Cancer 2016;63(6):973–82.

2. Borowitz MJ, Devidas M, Hunger SP, et al. Clinical significance of minimal resid-ual disease in childhood acute lymphoblastic leukemia and its relationship to other prognostic factors: a Children's Oncology Group study. Blood 2008; 111(12):5477–85.

3. Conter V, Bartram CR, Valsecchi MG, et al. Molecular response to treatment re-defines all prognostic factors in children and adolescents with B-cell precursor acute lymphoblastic leukemia: results in 3184 patients of the AIEOP-BFM ALL 2000 study. Blood 2010;115(16):3206–14.

4. Vora A, Goulden N, Wade R, et al. Treatment reduction for children and young adults with low-risk acute lymphoblastic leukaemia defined by minimal residual disease (UKALL 2003): a randomised controlled trial. Lancet Oncol 2013;14(3): 199–209.

5. Stow P, Key L, Chen X, et al. Clinical significance of low levels of minimal residual disease at the end of remission induction therapy in childhood acute lympho-blastic leukemia. Blood 2010;115(23):4657–63.

6. Leung W, Pui CH, Coustan-Smith E, et al. Detectable minimal residual disease before hematopoietic cell transplantation is prognostic but does not preclude cure for children with very-high-risk leukemia. Blood 2012;120(2):468–72.

7. Akabane H, Logan A. Clinical significance and management of MRD in adults with acute lymphoblastic leukemia. Clin Adv Hematol Oncol 2020;18(7):413–22.

8. Bruggemann M, Kotrova M. Minimal residual disease in adult ALL: technical as-pects and implications for correct clinical interpretation. Blood Adv 2017;1(25): 2456–66.

9. Cassaday RD, Stevenson PA, Wood BL, et al. Description and prognostic signif-icance of the kinetics of minimal residual disease status in adults with acute lymphoblastic leukemia treated with HyperCVAD. Am J Hematol 2018;93(4): 546–52.

10. O'Connor D, Moorman AV, Wade R, et al. Use of minimal residual disease assess-ment to redefine induction failure in pediatric acute lymphoblastic leukemia. J Clin Oncol 2017;35(6):660–7.

11. Gupta S, Devidas M, Loh ML, et al. Flow-cytometric vs. -morphologic assessment of remission in childhood acute lymphoblastic leukemia: a report from the Chil-dren's Oncology Group (COG). Leukemia 2018;32(6):1370–9.

12. Lucio P, Parreira A, van den Beemd MW, et al. Flow cytometric analysis of normal B cell differentiation: a frame of reference for the detection of minimal residual dis-ease in precursor-B-ALL. Leukemia 1999;13(3):419–27.

13. Shalabi H, Yuan CM, Kulshreshtha A, et al. Disease detection methodologies in relapsed B-cell acute lymphoblastic leukemia: opportunities for improvement. Pe-diatr Blood Cancer 2020;67(4):e28149.

14. Flohr T, Schrauder A, Cazzaniga G, et al. Minimal residual disease-directed risk stratification using real-time quantitative PCR analysis of immunoglobulin and T-cell receptor gene rearrangements in the international multicenter trial AIEOP-BFM ALL 2000 for childhood acute lymphoblastic leukemia. Leukemia 2008; 22(4):771–82.

15. Campana D. Determination of minimal residual disease in leukaemia patients. Br J Haematol 2003;121(6):823–38.

16. Gabert J, Beillard E, van der Velden VH, et al. Standardization and quality control studies of 'real-time' quantitative reverse transcriptase polymerase chain reaction of fusion gene transcripts for residual disease detection in leukemia - a Europe against Cancer program. Leukemia 2003;17(12):2318–57.

17. Faham M, Zheng J, Moorhead M, et al. Deep-sequencing approach for minimal residual disease detection in acute lymphoblastic leukemia. Blood 2012;120(26): 5173–80.

18. Pulsipher MA, Carlson C, Langholz B, et al. IgH-V(D)J NGS-MRD measurement pre- and early post-allotransplant defines very low- and very high-risk ALL patients. Blood 2015;125(22):3501–8.

19. Wood B, Wu D, Crossley B, et al. Measurable residual disease detection by high-throughput sequencing improves risk stratification for pediatric B-ALL. Blood 2018;131(12):1350–9.

20. Della Starza I, De Novi LA, Santoro A, et al. Digital droplet PCR and next-generation sequencing refine minimal residual disease monitoring in acute lymphoblastic leukemia. Leuk Lymphoma 2019;60(11):2838–40.

21. Della Starza I, Chiaretti S, De Propris MS, et al. Minimal residual disease in acute lymphoblastic leukemia: technical and clinical advances. Front Oncol 2019; 9:726.

22. Gaipa G, Cazzaniga G, Valsecchi MG, et al. Time point-dependent concordance of flow cytometry and real-time quantitative polymerase chain reaction for minimal residual disease detection in childhood acute lymphoblastic leukemia. Haematologica 2012;97(10):1582–93.

23. Tembhare PR, Subramanian PG, Ghogale S, et al. A high-sensitivity 10-color flow cytometric minimal residual disease assay in B-lymphoblastic leukemia/lymphoma can easily achieve the sensitivity of 2-in-10(6) and is superior to standard minimal residual disease assay: a study of 622 patients. Cytometry B Clin Cytom 2020;98(1):57–67.

24. Theunissen PMJ, Sedek L, De Haas V, et al. Detailed immunophenotyping of B-cell precursors in regenerating bone marrow of acute lymphoblastic leukaemia patients: implications for minimal residual disease detection. Br J Haematol 2017; 178(2):257–66.

25. Fossat C, Roussel M, Arnoux I, et al. Methodological aspects of minimal residual disease assessment by flow cytometry in acute lymphoblastic leukemia: a French multicenter study. Cytometry B Clin Cytom 2015;88(1):21–9.

26. Theunissen P, Mejstrikova E, Sedek L, et al. Standardized flow cytometry for highly sensitive MRD measurements in B-cell acute lymphoblastic leukemia. Blood 2017;129(3):347–57.

27. Schumich A, Maurer-Granofszky M, Attarbaschi A, et al. Flow-cytometric minimal residual disease monitoring in blood predicts relapse risk in pediatric B-cell precursor acute lymphoblastic leukemia in trial AIEOP-BFM-ALL 2000. Pediatr Blood Cancer 2019;66(5):e27590.

28. Pui CH, Pei D, Raimondi SC, et al. Clinical impact of minimal residual disease in children with different subtypes of acute lymphoblastic leukemia treated with Response-Adapted therapy. Leukemia 2017;31(2):333–9.

29. Chen X, Wood BL. Monitoring minimal residual disease in acute leukemia: technical challenges and interpretive complexities. Blood Rev 2017;31(2):63–75.

30. Shaver AC, Seegmiller AC. B lymphoblastic leukemia minimal residual disease assessment by flow cytometric analysis. Clin Lab Med 2017;37(4):771–85.

31. Keeney M, Halley JG, Rhoads DD, et al. Marked variability in reported minimal residual disease lower level of detection of 4 hematolymphoid neoplasms: a survey of participants in the College of American Pathologists Flow Cytometry Proficiency Testing Program. Arch Pathol Lab Med 2015;139(10):1276–80.

32. Keeney M, Wood BL, Hedley BD, et al. A QA program for MRD testing demonstrates that systematic education can reduce discordance among experienced interpreters. Cytometry B Clin Cytom 2018;94(2):239–49.
33. Hupp MM, Bashleben C, Cardinali JL, et al. Participation in the College of American Pathologists Laboratory accreditation program decreases variability in B-lymphoblastic leukemia and plasma cell myeloma flow cytometric minimal residual disease testing: a follow-up survey. Arch Pathol Lab Med 2021;145(3): 336–42.
34. Kroft SH, Harrington AM. Flow cytometry of B-Cell neoplasms. Clin Lab Med 2017;37(4):697–723.
35. Jain S, Mehta A, Kapoor G, et al. Evaluating new markers for minimal residual disease analysis by flow cytometry in precursor B lymphoblastic leukemia. Indian J Hematol Blood Transfus 2018;34(1):48–53.
36. Borowitz MJ, Pullen DJ, Winick N, et al. Comparison of diagnostic and relapse flow cytometry phenotypes in childhood acute lymphoblastic leukemia: implications for residual disease detection: a report from the children's oncology group. Cytometry B Clin Cytom 2005;68(1):18–24.
37. Cherian S, Miller V, McCullouch V, et al. A novel flow cytometric assay for detection of residual disease in patients with B-lymphoblastic leukemia/lymphoma post anti-CD19 therapy. Cytometry B Clin Cytom 2018;94(1):112–20.
38. Belkina AC, Ciccolella CO, Anno R, et al. Automated optimized parameters for T-distributed stochastic neighbor embedding improve visualization and analysis of large datasets. Nat Commun 2019;10(1):5415.
39. Mair F, Hartmann FJ, Mrdjen D, et al. The end of gating? An introduction to automated analysis of high dimensional cytometry data. Eur J Immunol 2016;46(1): 34–43.
40. Lucchesi S, Nolfi E, Pettini E, et al. Computational analysis of multiparametric flow cytometric data to dissect B cell subsets in vaccine studies. Cytometry A 2020; 97(3):259–67.
41. DiGiuseppe JA, Tadmor MD, Pe'er D. Detection of minimal residual disease in B lymphoblastic leukemia using viSNE. Cytometry B Clin Cytom 2015;88(5): 294–304.
42. Perfetto SP, Chattopadhyay PK, Roederer M. Seventeen-colour flow cytometry: unravelling the immune system. Nat Rev Immunol 2004;4(8):648–55.
43. Robinson JP. Spectral flow cytometry-Quo vadimus? Cytometry A 2019;95(8): 823–4.
44. Park LM, Lannigan J, Jaimes MC. OMIP-069: forty-color full spectrum flow cytometry panel for deep immunophenotyping of major cell subsets in human peripheral blood. Cytometry A 2020;97(10):1044–51.
45. Latis E, Michonneau D, Leloup C, et al. Cellular and molecular profiling of T-cell subsets at the onset of human acute GVHD. Blood Adv 2020;4(16):3927–42.

Artificial Intelligence in the Genetic Diagnosis of Rare Disease

Kiely N. James, PhD[a,1], Sujal Phadke, PhD[a,1],
Terence C. Wong, PhD[a,1], Shimul Chowdhury, PhD[b,1,*]

KEYWORDS

- Genomics • Precision medicine • Natural language processing
- Artificial intelligence

KEY POINTS

- The use of artificial intelligence can streamline the lengthy process currently required to clinically interpret a genome.
- Natural language processing can eliminate much of the human variability and bias that is involved in translating information from the medical record.
- Deep learning approaches can expedite the prioritization of genetic variants during interpretation of genomic data.
- The promise of genomic medicine will be fully realized only if the time and cost of analyzing genomic data continue to decrease.

INTRODUCTION

More than 7000 rare diseases have been described, with prevalence ranging from fewer than 1 in a million (eg, metachromatic leukodystrophy) to greater than 1 in 10,000 (eg, sickle cell anemia), and of these, approximately 70% are largely genetic in origin[1]. In total, an estimated 263 to 446 million individuals are thought to be afflicted by rare diseases worldwide[1]. The identification of causal genetic variants in these individuals enables patient-specific clinical management, referred to as genomic or precision medicine, which has the potential to improve patient survival and quality of life, and reduce health care costs[2,3].

This article originally appeared in *Advances in Molecular Pathology*, Volume 3, Issue 1, November 2020.
a Genomics, Rady Children's Institute for Genomic Medicine, 7910 Frost Street, MC5129, San Diego, CA 92123, USA; b Rady Children's Institute for Genomic Medicine, 7910 Frost Street, MC5129, San Diego, CA 92123, USA
1 All authors contributed equally to this work.
* Corresponding author.
E-mail address: schowdhury@rchsd.org

Genetic diagnosis is achieved through testing of specific genes or by more comprehensive interrogation via whole exome sequencing (WES) or whole genome sequencing (WGS; **Box 1**). The typical workflow for diagnostic genomic sequencing in affected individuals involves sample collection and processing, phenotypic evaluation, genetic variant detection, genetic variant interpretation, and reporting (**Fig. 1**). In cases in which the pretest differential diagnosis is narrow and pathognomonic features are present, a single gene or gene panel test is likely to be ordered. However, the use of clinical WES and WGS is growing more widespread as costs and turn-around-times drop. In both methods, primary phenotypes are used during genomic analysis to inform gene review and variant prioritization based on the overlap of canonical disease descriptions with the patient's phenotype, a necessary step, as WES and WGS can produce approximately 25,000 genetic variants and upward of 4 to 5 million variants, respectively[4].

Artificial intelligence (AI) has the potential to transform many aspects of the practice of medicine, including rare disease diagnosis. Defined as the ability of a computer or machine to perform tasks that are normally associated with human intelligence, AI can

---

Box 1
Glossary of Key Terms

Bayesian Probability Model: probability expressed as a degree of belief in an event based on prior knowledge about the event, such as the results of previous experiments[40].

Computer Vision: a subfield of artificial intelligence concerned with understanding, analyzing, and interpreting visual images

Deep Learning: a branch of machine learning that combines large multilayered neural networks with large computing power to learn and recognize patterns

Electronic Health Record: a digital version of a patient's medical chart over time, including medical history, diagnoses, medications, treatment plans, immunizations, radiology images, and laboratory and genetic test results

Machine Learning: a subfield of artificial intelligence concerned with developing computer algorithms to learn from data, identify patterns, and build models without predefined assumptions

Natural Language Processing: a subfield of artificial intelligence concerned with understanding, analyzing, and interpreting human language

Neural Network: a statistical model used in machine learning based on neurons in the human brain to process data through multiple layers, with adaptive weights tuned to optimize results.

Ontology: a representation of entities and the relationships between them, often visualized as nodes connected by labeled paths. Example: in the Human Phenotype Ontology, the node/term "Short stature" is connected to its parent node/term "Abnormality of height" by the path "is a"

Random Forest: a machine learning algorithm that outputs the mode or median of multiple decision trees for classification. This aggregation protects against overfitting to training datasets

Random Walk: a machine learning algorithm that involves random sampling from large amounts of data to iteratively pinpoint which sources to use for classification

Whole Exome Sequencing: the process of determining the sequence of the coding regions of the genome. This is approximately 1% to 2% of the entire genome.

Whole Genome Sequencing: the process of determining the complete DNA sequence of an individual

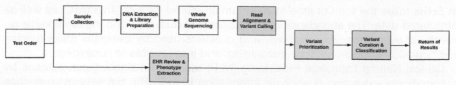

Fig. 1. Typical genome sequencing workflow to diagnose genetic diseases. A test order is placed for genomic sequencing and a biological sample is collected. For rare genetic disease, blood is often the preferred sample type. DNA is extracted from blood and sequencing libraries are prepared. Genomic sequencing is performed and the resulting sequencing reads are aligned to the reference human genome and variants are called. In parallel, phenotypic features are extracted from a patient's EHR and translated into phenotypic terms. Annotated variants and phenotypic terms are integrated to identify genetic variants that are the likely cause of disease. These variants are curated, classified according to standard guidelines, and reported to the clinical team. Phenotype extraction and variant prioritization (highlighted in *orange*) can potentially be automated with the use of computational or artificial intelligence methods. Note that read alignment and variant calling (highlighted in *blue*) typically incorporates AI methods to achieve an increased sensitivity and specificity[39]. Variant curation and classification (highlighted in *blue*) is another area in which AI may prove helpful.

be divided into subfields, such as natural language processing, machine learning (including neural networks and deep learning), computer vision (including image recognition), and cognitive computing (see **Box 1**). Since its initial development in the 1950s, AI has achieved more widespread use in recent decades due to decreased data storage costs, advances in computer algorithms, and gains in computing power. Through its ability to analyze increasingly large amounts of data in an unbiased manner, AI has been applied to improve patient outcomes through more accurate diagnoses and more comprehensive monitoring[5].

In the field of rare and ultra-rare disease, the use of AI may help overcome the limits of human experience-based reasoning and reduce the time needed to reach a diagnosis. Because there are many rare genetic disorders, clinicians may have never seen a particular genetic disorder before encountering it in their patient. Here, we review the current landscape of AI platforms for phenotype extraction and phenotype-driven variant prioritization in WGS for the diagnosis of rare disease. Currently, automatic phenotypic extraction from the electronic health record (EHR) is quite rare, whereas the use of phenotype-aware automated variant prioritization tools is fairly common. We survey the available tools for both processes, highlight strengths and weaknesses, and provide examples of their application in the clinical setting. Finally, we end with a discussion of the limitations and challenges of AI-assisted diagnosis of rare disease and considerations of confidentiality and security related to genomic data.

SIGNIFICANCE
Artificial Intelligence in Phenotype Extraction

Linking phenotypes to known genetic disease descriptions is essential for diagnosis. The primary source of clinical phenotypic information is the EHR, which collects granular, individual-level clinical information. EHRs have been widely implemented in most major hospital systems to meet regulatory and billing requirements. EHRs present a comprehensive, quantitative portrait of the patient's observed symptoms and signs as well as additional information including ongoing or resolved prior diagnoses, medical and surgical history, family history, birth history, medications, interventions and responses, laboratory tests, and diagnostic investigations. The medical data contained in EHRs takes the form of time-stamped unstructured data or "free text," as well as structured data. The abundance of unstructured textual data and the remarkable diversity of synonyms, abbreviations, and qualifiers used by clinicians make manual EHR curation error-prone, time-consuming, and inaccessible to nonexperts.

Clinical Natural Language Processing (NLP) tools can mitigate these burdens by automatically extracting phenotypic information from EHRs, but several challenges have slowed their adoption. In addition to privacy concerns regarding storage or use of EHR data (see *Limitations and Challenges*), the matching of both structured and unstructured EHR data to potential diagnoses or genes requires translation across vocabularies or ontologies that were not expressly designed to be linked. Two forms of structured data commonly present in EHRs are International Classification of Diseases (ICD) codes, which represent diagnoses and are used mainly for billing purposes, and Systematized Nomenclature of Medicine (SNOMED) terms, which represent clinical findings and were developed to allow for precise, controlled information sharing among clinicians caring for a patient (**Table 1**). Unstructured EHR data must be extracted into some structured format, such as Unified Medical Language System (UMLS) concepts, Human Phenotype Ontology (HPO), and SNOMED Clinical Terms (SNOMED CT), or Current Procedural Terminology (CPT) and ICD codes, often sorted by frequency or probability (**Fig. 2**, **Table 2**). In addition, tools such as the Monarch Initiative can be used to map between different ontologies. Variant prioritization tools accept phenotypic data in specific formats, most commonly HPO (**Table 3**). Some tools for automated phenotype extraction include a mapping step to translate phenotype terms from other ontologies or vocabularies into HPO terms, but robust tools for this translation step are still needed. In this context, the Monarch Initiative promises to fill an important unmet need to leverage semantic relationships between biological concepts by developing key ontological resources to harmonize phenotype ontologies in the Unified Phenotype Ontology[6]. The Monarch Initiative uses uPheno (http://obofoundry.org/ontology/upheno) to find candidate genes and potential animal models for human diseases. Allowing for inexact matching during intervocabulary translation while retaining accuracy and high information content remains an important challenge[7].

Multiple clinical NLP solutions are available for extraction of phenotypic information. A representative sample is reviewed in **Table 2**.

Unified Medical Language System–based clinical Natural Language Processing tools
UMLS, which is a collection of several controlled vocabularies in biomedical sciences, provides a base mapping structure for 2 popular clinical NLP tools: MetaMap and Clinical Text Analysis and Knowledge Extraction System (cTAKES)[8].

- *MetaMap:* MetaMap (https://metamap.nlm.nih.gov/) is a public resource developed by the National Library of Medicine to extract and standardize biomedical text to medical concepts in UMLS[9]. It integrates knowledge-intensive approach and computational linguistic techniques. MetaMap uses a nonstandard input text that is frequently found in the form of MEDLINE/PubMed citations. For each phrase in input text, MetaMap produces default output as a human-readable list of candidate Metathesaurus concepts matching or part of the phrase.
- *cTAKES*: cTAKES combines the UMLS framework with the OpenNLP natural language processing toolkit to offer an open-source NLP system that extracts clinical information from unstructured data in clinical notes[10]. cTAKES accepts either plain text or clinical document architecture—compliant XML documents as input. cTAKES is a modular system of pipelined components combining rule-based and machine learning algorithms. cTAKES is available at http://www.ohnlp.org/.

Table 1
Ontologies Used in Natural Language Processing/Artificial Intelligence Tools for Genetic Diagnosis

Abbreviation	Ontology	Description	References
DO	Disease Ontology	Hierarchy of disease descriptions, with embedded information about inheritance patterns and OMIM phenotype terms.	Schriml et al[41], 2019
GO	Gene Ontology	Loosely hierarchical computational model of biological systems, which includes 3 sub-ontologies: GO-BP (biological process), GO-CC (cellular component), GO-MF (molecular function).	Ashburner et al[22], 2000
HPO	Human Phenotype Ontology	Collaboratively developed hierarchical ontology, originally based on OMIM disease descriptions. Terms are connected by "is-a" (ie, subset) relationships.	Köhler et al[42], 2019
ICD	International Classification of Diseases	Set of alphanumeric codes representing diagnoses, with some characters optional for specifying body regions, etiology or severity. Used for medical billing and research; maintained by the World Health Organization.	World Health Organization[43], 2004
OMIM	Online Mendelian Inheritance in Man	Catalog of human diseases and their genetic causes.	McKusick-Nathans Institute of Genetic Medicine[44]
SNOMED	Systematized Nomenclature of Medicine	Large collaboratively developed medical vocabulary used for precise recording and sharing of clinical information. Merger of 2 ontologies, developed by the College of American Pathologists and the UK's National Health Service (NHS).	Cornet & de Keizer[45], 2008
UMLS	Unified Medical Language System	A set of tools for translating between clinical and biomedical vocabularies including SNOMED and ICD. Maintained by the US National Library of Medicine.	Bodenreider[38], 2004
uPheno	The Unified Phenotype Ontology	A key resource to map and harmonize between various ontologies and facilitate discovery of candidate genes and potential animal models for human diseases. Developed and maintained by The Monarch Initiative.	Mungall et al[46], 2017

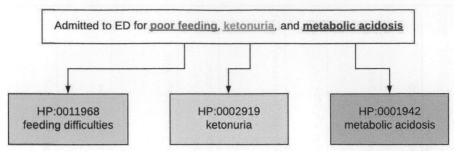

Fig. 2. Extraction and translation of phenotypes from EHRs to ontology terms. Automated NLP methods can be used to extract a patient's phenotypes from the EHR and translate them into a standardized vocabulary in an ontology, such as HPO.

Human Phenotype Ontology–based clinical Natural Language Processing tools
The HPO is an atlas of standardized vocabulary of phenotypic abnormalities reported in human disease with the aim of facilitating phenotype-driven differential diagnostics, genomic diagnostics, and translational research. NLP tools such as ClinPhen, use HPO as a phenotype mapping structure for clinical phenotypes. In addition, tools such as Phenolyzer or Phenomizer (not discussed) can take HPO terms and create patient-specific gene lists to help guide genomic analysis[11,12].

- *ClinPhen*: ClinPhen (http://bejerano.stanford.edu/clinphen/) is a fast, easy-to-use, high-precision, and high-sensitivity tool that scans through free-text notes in a patient's clinical notes and returns a prioritized list of patient phenotypes using HPO terms[13]. These phenotypes can be input to gene ranking tools that rank the causative gene for Mendelian diseases. ClinPhen uses hash tables created from sentences, subsentences, and words in clinical notes. It was benchmarked as performing 20 times faster than cTAKES and MetaMap[14].

Semi-supervised clustering-based clinical Natural Language Processing tools
Semi-supervised approaches to phenotypic extraction integrate prior knowledge with cluster analyses to generate a priority or rank list of phenotypes to aid clinical diagnostics.

- *DAPS:* Denoising Autoencoders for Phenotype Stratification (DAPS; https://github.com/greenelab/DAPS) is a machine learning algorithm that uses semi-supervised technique for exploring phenotypes in the EHR. The algorithm is trained using clustering via principal components analysis and t-distributed stochastic neighbor embedding[15]. A typical output includes a list of cosegregating phenotypes describing distinct disease conditions.
- *PheCap*: PheCAP uses a semi-supervised approach to automated extraction of phenotypes from clinical notes[16]. PheCap accepts high-throughput structured and unstructured data from the EHR and produces a phenotype algorithm, the probability of the phenotype for all patients, and a binary (yes or no) phenotype classification. PheCAP suffers in being substantially slower in performance than other tools such as ClinPhen and CLiX ENRICH[16].

Systematized Nomenclature of Medicine Clinical Terms–based clinical Natural Language Processing tools
SNOMED CT is a comprehensive and multilingual health terminology standard developed to assist electronic exchange of clinical health information. It is also a required standard in interoperability specifications of the US Healthcare Information

Table 2
Clinical Natural Language Processing Tools for Phenotypic Extraction

Tool	Artificial Intelligence	Input	Output	References
MetaMap	Unsupervised approaches for automatic indexing to map medical text to Metathesaurus concepts, unsupervised approaches to automatic disambiguation of Metathesaurus concepts (also called as Word Sense Disambiguation)	Unstructured and structured data from electronic health record (EHR)	Human-readable and machine-readable list of candidate Metathesaurus concepts in MetaMap machine output (MMO), XML and colorized MetaMap formats	Aronson & Lang[9], 2010
cTAKES (2010)	Rule-based and machine learning algorithms used to generate outputs	Unstructured and structured data from EHR	Machine-readable XMI CAS file including annotations for anatomic sites, signs and symptoms, medical procedures, diseases/disorders and medications, normalized Unified Medical Language System concept unique identifiers, uncertainty score and patient specific	Savova et al[10], 2010
ClinPhen	Rule-based sentence analysis process	Unstructured and structured data from EHR	Machine-readable hash tables created from sentences, subsentences, and words, human-readable sorted list of all Human Phenotype Ontology (HPO) phenotypes found, with the most frequent- and earliest-appearing phenotypes at the top	Deisseroth et al[13], 2019

(continued on next page)

Table 2
(continued)

Tool	Artificial Intelligence	Input	Output	References
DAPS	Machine learning used for training	Unstructured and structured data from EHR	Human and machine-readable list of cosegregating phenotypes describing distinct disease conditions	Beaulieu-Jones & Greene[15], 2016, https://github.com/greenelab/DAPS
PheCap	Semi-supervised approach used in phenotype extraction	Unstructured and structured data from EHR	Human-readable and machine-readable probability of the phenotype for a patient, a binary phenotype classification (yes or no)	Zhang et al[16], 2019
CliniThink	Proprietary artificial intelligence technology to parse EHR Data into Systemized Nomenclature of Medicine (SNOMED) terms	Unstructured and structured data from EHR	List of SNOMED terms; optional step to map SNOMED to HPO terms	Clark et al[17], 2019

Table 3
Phenotype-Driven Variant Prioritization Tools

Tool (Year)	Artificial Intelligence	Input	Output	References
eXtasy (2013)	Machine learning training (random forests)	VCF + HPO terms	Annotated variant list including phenotype-derived gene-level rank	Aerts et al[19], 2006 & Sifrim et al[20], 2013
Phevor (2014)	Ontological propagation algorithm used to assess likelihood of gene involvement in disease (including for novel genes)	Ranked variant list (eg, VAAST format) + HPO/DO/GO/ OMIM terms	Re-ranked variant list	Singleton et al[21], 2014
Phen-Gen (2014)	Machine learning (Random walk with restart algorithm) used for phenotype (ie, disease) risk estimation. Bayesian framework integrates patient genetic and phenotypic risk estimates.	VCF + HPO terms + pedigree (PED) file	Ranked gene list (for genes present on input VCF) and separate file of annotated variants from those genes	Javed et al[24], 2014
Exomiser (2015)	Machine learning (random walk algorithm) used for novel disease gene discovery mode (ExomeWalker)	VCF + HPO/OMIM/DECIPHER/ ORDO terms	VCF: ranked variant list HTML: ranked gene list with associated diseases and variants in the gene embedded, in HTML format	Smedley et al[26], 2015
Xrare (2019)	Machine learning (gradient boosting decision tree algorithm) used to generate gene-phenotype scores and to train the Xrare variant classifier	VCF + HPO terms	Ranked variant list	Li et al[18], 2019

(continued on next page)

Table 3
(continued)

Tool (Year)	Artificial Intelligence	Input	Output	References
DeepPVP (2019)	Deep neural network used for training and variant classification	VCF + HPO terms	Ranked variant list	Boudellioua et al[27], 2019
eDiva (2019)	Machine learning (random forest model) used for variant pathogenicity prediction (eDiva-Score) eDiva-Prioritize: incorporates HPO term similarity scoring underlying the Phenomizer tool (see Kohler et al)	VCF + HPO terms	Ranked variant list	Bosio et al[28], 2019 Kohler et al [25], 2009
Moon (2019)	Bayesian framework combines gene-phenotype similarity score and variant pathogenicity scores	VCF + HPO terms	Ranked variant list	Clark et al[17], 2019

Abbreviations: DECIPHER, DatabasE of genomiC varIation and Phenotype in Humans using Ensembl Resources; DO, Disease Ontology; GO, Gene Ontology; HPO, Human Phenotype Ontology; OMIM, Online Inheritance in Man; VAAST, ORDO, Orphanet Rare Disease Ontology; Variant Annotation, Analysis and Search Tool; VCF, variant call format.

Technology Standards Panel. SNOMED CT can be mapped to other coding systems including ICD-9 and ICD-10 to facilitate semantic interoperability. CliniThink is a leading phenotype extraction platform that primarily uses SNOMED CT ontologies.

- *CliniThink*: The CliniThink platform CLiX ENRICH uses SNOMED CT for phenotypic extraction. The proprietary CLiX (Corporate Learning and Information Exchange) system encodes clinical free text (pre-coordinated) to enrich for SNOMED dictionary terms and select contextually correct SNOMED concepts (post-coordinated). The standard output from CLiX ENRICH is in the form of SNOMED CT that includes diagnosis, medication, sign/symptoms, and contextual concepts, such as historical reference and negation[17].

Artificial Intelligence in Phenotype-Driven Variant Prioritization

As WES began to become more widely available as a clinical test approximately 2012 to 2015, numerous groups developed tools to aid in the evaluation of the large number of genomic variants generated per case. Many recent variant prioritization tools have incorporated AI methods into their training and implementation, and a subset uses patient phenotype information input to rank variants in a phenotype-driven manner. Several AI methods have emerged as of particular importance for these tools:

- Machine learning during tool training with positive and negative control variant datasets to optimize sensitivity and specificity
- Incorporation of multiple gene interactomes and similarity metrics to enable disease prediction for novel genes
- Calculation of a similarity score between the patient phenotype and gene or disease phenotypes, often relying on one or more phenotypic ontology

The exact format of the phenotypic input required has varied among variant prioritization tools as the clinical genomics field has co-opted multiple biological and clinical ontologies such as Gene Ontology (GO), ICD, HPO, Disease Ontology (DO), and Online Mendelian Inheritance in Man (OMIM), with recent convergence on HPO as a consensus input vocabulary (see **Tables 1** and **3**). Most variant prioritization tools developed to date were designed and tested with manual input of phenotypic terms. To scale with the ongoing increase in demand for clinical next-generation sequencing (NGS), variant prioritization tools will need to be optimized to accept phenotypic terms that are automatically extracted from medical records[18].

First-Generation Phenotype-Based Variant Prioritization Tools

A first generation of phenotype-based variant prioritization tools for NGS was published in 2013 to 2014. All accepted HPO terms as input, but some also accepted phenotypic terms in other formats, reflecting the lack of early consensus on a phenotypic ontology.

- *EXtasy*: One of the first published phenotype-driven variant prioritization tools, EXtasy was trained on positive and negative control variant datasets using a random forest algorithm, a form of machine learning. EXtasy incorporates patient phenotype data input as HPO terms to derive a gene-level metric, which is integrated with metrics of variant pathogenicity to rank variants in a phenotype-driven manner[19,20]. The gene-level metric integrates information about disease phenotypes and gene function, similarity and interaction from multiple sources including biomedical literature, GO functional annotation (see **Table 1**), gene expression datasets, and protein interactomes. This tool's reliance on machine learning for training and integration of multiple data sources for gene-disease modeling was prescient of approaches that have become widely adopted.

- *Phevor*: In Phevor, patient phenotypic terms are input together with annotated variants, to a propagation algorithm, which transmits weighted values across and within several biomedical ontologies containing information about relationships between phenotypic features (HPO, DO, Mammalian Phenotype Ontology) or about gene function and interaction (GO)[21]. Earlier work linking HPO terms to genes and genes to GO terms allows for propagation between phenotypic and gene ontologies[22,23]. Ultimately the output of Phevor's propagation algorithm is a re-scoring of candidate variants, ranked by a combination of relevance to patient phenotype and predicted pathogenicity. Phevor's algorithm was shown to detect (ie, highly rank) variants in novel disease genes, an important marker of the algorithm's utility for gene discovery[21].
- *Phen-Gen*: Phen-Gen uses a Bayesian framework (see **Box 1**) to generate gene-level estimations of disease involvement based on patient phenotype and variant data, using an implementation of Phenomizer[24]. Phenomizer is a tool that calculates similarity scores between HPO input queries and genetic diseases that have been annotated with HPO terms[25].
- *Exomiser*: Exomiser can be run in several modes, depending on whether the goal is to search for variants in known or novel disease genes[26]. One mode, Exome-Walker, uses a random walk algorithm within a protein interactome, seeded by genes input by the user, to search for novel disease genes. Another mode, PhenIX, uses a similar phenotype ranking approach to that used by PhenoDB: known disease genes are scored for likelihood of disease involvement based on similarity of the input patient phenotype terms to those in OMIM disease entries; then the gene-level score is combined with variant pathogenicity scoring to generate an overall variant ranking.

Second-Generation Phenotype-Based Variant Prioritization Tools

Several new phenotype-based variant prioritization tools were published in 2019, including Xrare, DeepPVP, eDiva, and Moon. These tools showcase the increasing integration of machine learning, including use of neural networks (DeepPVP). All of these tools accept HPO terms as input, perhaps reflecting growing consensus in the field for adoption of that ontology.

- *Xrare*: The development of Xrare incorporated a gradient-boosting decision tree (GBDT) algorithm, a form of machine learning that can robustly handle redundant, highly correlated inputs, for training[18]. The GBDT approach was also used to generate the model's gene-phenotype scores, seeded by genes with known phenotypes. The gene-phenotype scores are static scores determined for each gene-phenotype pair, calculated using 10 gene interactomes, among them the 3 GO sub-ontologies (see **Table 1**), BLAST for sequence similarity, and Reactome for shared pathways[18]. This gene-phenotype score is combined with variant-level features such as allele frequency, gene constraint and in silico variant pathogenicity predictions, to rank input variants. Xrare also includes a phenotype similarity measure developed to handle noisy, imprecise patient phenotypic data and compare it to phenotype sets associated with disease or genes within its model. Xrare is notable for its consideration of input data imprecision and redundancy, which will likely prove important in the development of tools designed to accept phenotypic data automatically generated from EMRs.

- *DeepPVP*: DeepPVP uses a deep neural network to classify variants (see **Box 1**)[27]. Similar to Xrare and Exomiser-PhenIX, DeepPVP scores genes for similarity between their associated phenotypes (drawn from multiple databases spanning animal model results, gene expression data, and GO) (see **Table 1**) and the input patient phenotype, both of which are instantiated by sets of HPO terms[27]. This similarity score is one of the features input to the neural network–based variant classifier.

- *eDiva*: The training of eDiva's variant pathogenicity classifier, eDiva-Score, used a random forest machine learning approach[28]. A downstream module, eDiva-Prioritize, relies on an HPO similarity scoring metric built on the Phenomizer tool (as does Phen-Gen's phenotype-driven risk estimate; see **Table 3**) to compute similarity between patient phenotype and the disease association of genes.

- *Moon*: Moon computes a similarity score between the patient's phenotype term set and many disease-specific phenotype term sets to rank diseases by likelihood[17]. An interesting innovation by Moon is that the disease-specific phenotype term sets are generated using NLP of the medical literature, as opposed to, for example, OMIM-derived phenotype term lists used by other prioritization tools. A Bayesian model combines this disease likelihood ranking with variant pathogenicity scores derived from numerous sources.

DISCUSSION/SUMMARY
Limitations and Challenges

The promise of AI and the potential benefits it could provide to a health care system[29] have led to a large number of research studies demonstrating AI's applications in various fields of medicine[30], including its application in genomics and precision medicine[17,31,32]. However, the vast majority of these studies have been performed retrospectively, testing against already performed expert interpretation[30]. In addition, robust randomized control trials are limited in assessing AI-based approaches compared with current clinical practice. Thus, the true impact and implementation of AI in genomic interpretation has not yet been realized.

Recent review articles have framed the current challenges of AI in medicine[33] as well as the challenges associated with the clinical interpretation of genomic data more broadly[34]. The current bottlenecks of time-intensive clinical variant interpretation, and the lack of qualified experts to clinically interpret genomic data continue to hinder the widespread adoption of AI implementation in genomic analysis.

Current Challenges and Barriers to Address

- *Privacy*: Privacy issues related to genomic analysis remain regardless of the incorporation of AI-based approaches[35]. Genomic testing is highly sensitive (https://www.genome.gov/about-genomics/policy-issues/Privacy)   in   part because: (1) it can be interpreted as "identifiable information," (2) the potential for genomic analysis to reveal findings not related to the patient's current phenotype (incidental findings), and (3) potential impact to family members if pathogenic variants are inherited. The use of AI and the introduction of new applications into the genomic data analysis process requires careful consideration to ensure the tools and processes respect and protect patient privacy.

- *Human Resistance*: The field of genetics and genomics has traditionally been shepherded by clinical genetics and laboratory genetics professionals. However, as genomics becomes applied to all areas of medicine, the ability to allow other subspecialties and individuals with different backgrounds and training will be essential to scale genomic sequencing to all the patients that may benefit from this testing. Currently, there are approximately 5000 genetic counselors and 1500 clinical geneticists in the United States, numbers well below what would be required to deploy broader genomic sequencing (https://www.nsgc.org/). Thus, technology-based solutions will be required to serve the patient base for genomic sequencing that may benefit from this technology.

- *Lack of Regulation and Quality Control*: The vast majority of genetic tests fall under the category of laboratory developed tests that are governed and regulated by accreditation bodies such as the Clinical Laboratory Improvement Amendment and the College of American Pathologists. However, there are no current guidance for the validation and implementation of AI in the diagnosis of genetic disease, and the question of what is the right regulatory framework for AI remains unresolved[36]. The regulatory considerations for these novel approaches and technologies must be addressed before AI can be widely adopted across laboratories. There is a lack of published studies on AI implementation within genetic diagnostic pipelines. A collaborative, cross-laboratory effort to establish best practices for AI implementation in genetic testing would be valuable.

- *Lack of Gold Standard Truth Sets*: Genomic sequencing has benefited from the establishment of gold standard truth sets to assess the validity of genomic data generated via NGS[37]. Standards to assess the interpretation and clinical reporting of genomic data lag behind these sequencing validation truth sets, and will be required to allow laboratories to benchmark AI-based approaches.

- *Phenotypic Complexity*: Many diseases manifest as multiple phenotypes with variable severity, necessitating modeling of the phenotypic spectrum through NLP to facilitate (1) identification of core symptoms of the disease, (2) delineation of disease subtypes, (3) refinement of differential diagnoses, and (4) discovery of new genetic and pathophysiological mechanisms through hypothesis-driven research.

One Laboratory's Experience with Artificial Intelligence and Genetic Disease

In Clark and colleagues[17], the Rady Children's Institute for Genomic Medicine conducted a pilot study in which automated clinical NLP phenotype extraction from the EHR was performed, and that phenotypic information was then automatically incorporated into the rapid WGS analysis. Various steps in this process required thorough testing and development. Challenges included (1) thorough testing and validation on real patient data with genetic diagnoses at each step in the process; (2) the mappings of SNOMED CT and HPO were incomplete; (3) the accuracy of the NLP approach had to be thoroughly assessed; (4) the large phenotypic output (20 times greater than manual curation) had to be incorporated into the genomic analysis pipeline to prioritize a genetic diagnosis. The pilot pipeline achieved very strong concordance with expert manual interpretation (97% recall and 99% precision in 95 children with 97 genetic diseases) in retrospective cases. The investigators showed a proof of concept of how NLP and AI could aid in the rapid genetic diagnosis of children in the intensive care unit.

Final Thoughts

AI holds the potential to not just aid in the analysis of genomic data, but potentially in other areas of genomic medicine, including patient selection criteria and delivery of treatment guidance to maximize the utility of genomic sequencing (**Fig. 3**). To maximize the potential that genomic medicine has promised, the ability to deliver genetic diagnoses in a timeframe conducive to impacting clinical management is essential.

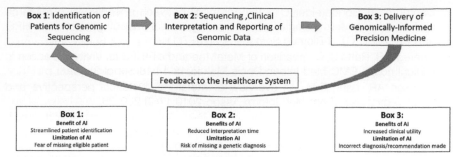

Fig. 3. Described are 3 major areas in which AI could advance and benefit genomic medicine with a continuous feedback loop as part of a learning health care system. One potential benefit and 1 potential limitation is described for each box.

Currently, many individuals with rare disease, who stand to benefit from genomic testing, lack access to it. Meanwhile, sequencing technologies continue to develop and drop in cost. Thus, the ability to comprehensively and efficiently analyze genomic data must maintain pace with sequencing improvements to ensure laboratories can meet the demand for genomic testing. The use of AI to aid genomic diagnosis presents a unique opportunity to address many of the current challenges and barriers that exist today, including the dearth of laboratory geneticists and trained workforce, and the cost and effort required to analyze genomic data. AI can help foster collaboration between academia and industry to ensure rapid developments in this evolving field. Realizing the potential of AI to aid genomic diagnosis will require a collaborative effort from the entire genomics community to ensure that these technologies can be deployed in a robust and responsible manner.

DISCLOSURE

This study was supported by grant U19HD077693, U01TR002271, UL1TR002550 from NICHD and NHGRI and NCATS.

REFERENCES

1. Nguengang Wakap S, Lambert DM, Olry A, et al. Estimating cumulative point prevalence of rare diseases: analysis of the Orphanet database. Eur J Hum Genet 2020;28(2):165–73.
2. Farnaes L, Hildreth A, Sweeney NM, et al. Rapid whole-genome sequencing decreases infant morbidity and cost of hospitalization. NPJ Genom Med 2018; 3(1):10.
3. Melbourne Genomics Health Alliance, Stark Z, Lunke S, et al. Meeting the challenges of implementing rapid genomic testing in acute pediatric care. Genet Med 2018;20(12):1554–63.
4. Kingsmore SF, Cakici JA, Clark MM, et al. A randomized, controlled trial of the analytic and diagnostic performance of singleton and trio, rapid genome and exome sequencing in ill infants. Am J Hum Genet 2019;105(4):719–33.
5. Brasil S, Pascoal C, Francisco R, et al. Artificial Intelligence (AI) in rare diseases: is the future brighter? Genes 2019;10(12):978.
6. Shefchek KA, Harris NL, Gargano M, et al. The Monarch Initiative in 2019: an integrative data and analytic platform connecting phenotypes to genotypes across species. Nucleic Acids Res 2020;48(D1):D704–15.

7. Dhombres F, Bodenreider O. Interoperability between phenotypes in research and healthcare terminologies—Investigating partial mappings between HPO and SNOMED CT. J Biomed Semantics 2016;7(1):3.

8. Reátegui R, Ratté S. Comparison of MetaMap and cTAKES for entity extraction in clinical notes. BMC Med Inform Decis Mak 2018 14;18(Suppl 3):74.

9. Aronson AR, Lang F-M. An overview of MetaMap: historical perspective and recent advances. J Am Med Inform Assoc 2010;17(3):229–36.

10. Savova GK, Masanz JJ, Ogren PV, et al. Mayo clinical Text Analysis and Knowledge Extraction System (cTAKES): architecture, component evaluation and applications. J Am Med Inform Assoc 2010;17(5):507–13.

11. Yang H, Robinson PN, Wang K. Phenolyzer: phenotype-based prioritization of candidate genes for human diseases. Nat Methods 2015;12(9):841–3.

12. Ullah MZ, Aono M, Seddiqui MH. Estimating a ranked list of human hereditary diseases for clinical phenotypes by using weighted bipartite network. Conf Proc IEEE Eng Med Biol Soc 2013;2013:3475–8.

13. Deisseroth CA, Birgmeier J, Bodle EE, et al. ClinPhen extracts and prioritizes patient phenotypes directly from medical records to expedite genetic disease diagnosis. Genet Med 2019;21(7):1585–93.

14. Liu C, Ta CN, Rogers JR, et al. Ensembles of natural language processing systems for portable phenotyping solutions. J Biomed Inform 2019;100:103318.

15. Beaulieu-Jones BK, Greene CS. Semi-supervised learning of the electronic health record for phenotype stratification. J Biomed Inform 2016;64:168–78.

16. Zhang Y, Cai T, Yu S, et al. High-throughput phenotyping with electronic medical record data using a common semi-supervised approach (PheCAP). Nat Protoc 2019;14(12):3426–44.

17. Clark MM, Hildreth A, Batalov S, et al. Diagnosis of genetic diseases in seriously ill children by rapid whole-genome sequencing and automated phenotyping and interpretation. Sci Transl Med 2019;11(489):eaat6177.

18. Li Q, Zhao K, Bustamante CD, et al. Xrare: a machine learning method jointly modeling phenotypes and genetic evidence for rare disease diagnosis. Genet Med 2019;21(9):2126–34.

19. Aerts S, Lambrechts D, Maity S, et al. Gene prioritization through genomic data fusion. Nat Biotechnol 2006;24(5):537–44.

20. Sifrim A, Popovic D, Tranchevent L-C, et al. eXtasy: variant prioritization by genomic data fusion. Nat Methods 2013;10(11):1083–4.

21. Singleton MV, Guthery SL, Voelkerding KV, et al. Phevor combines multiple biomedical ontologies for accurate identification of disease-causing alleles in single individuals and small nuclear families. Am J Hum Genet 2014;94(4):599–610.

22. Ashburner M, Ball CA, Blake JA, et al. Gene ontology: tool for the unification of biology. The Gene Ontology Consortium. Nat Genet 2000;25(1):25–9.

23. Robinson PN, Köhler S, Bauer S, et al. The human phenotype ontology: a tool for annotating and analyzing human hereditary disease. Am J Hum Genet 2008; 83(5):610–5.

24. Javed A, Agrawal S, Ng PC. Phen-Gen: combining phenotype and genotype to analyze rare disorders. Nat Methods 2014;11(9):935–7.

25. Köhler S, Schulz MH, Krawitz P, et al. Clinical diagnostics in human genetics with semantic similarity searches in ontologies. Am J Hum Genet 2009;85(4):457–64.

26. Smedley D, Jacobsen JOB, Jäger M, et al. Next-generation diagnostics and disease-gene discovery with the Exomiser. Nat Protoc 2015;10(12):2004–15.

27. Boudellioua I, Kulmanov M, Schofield PN, et al. DeepPVP: phenotype-based prioritization of causative variants using deep learning. BMC Bioinformatics 2019; 20(1):65.
28. Bosio M, Drechsel O, Rahman R, et al. eDiVA—Classification and prioritization of pathogenic variants for clinical diagnostics. Hum Mutat 2019;40(7):865–78.
29. Bodenheimer T, Sinsky C. From triple to quadruple aim: care of the patient requires care of the provider. Ann Fam Med 2014;12(6):573–6.
30. Kelly CJ, Karthikesalingam A, Suleyman M, et al. Key challenges for delivering clinical impact with artificial intelligence. BMC Med 2019;17(1):195.
31. Xu J, Yang P, Xue S, et al. Translating cancer genomics into precision medicine with artificial intelligence: applications, challenges and future perspectives. Hum Genet 2019;138(2):109–24.
32. Uddin M, Wang Y, Woodbury-Smith M. Artificial intelligence for precision medicine in neurodevelopmental disorders. NPJ Digit Med 2019;2(1):112.
33. Yu K-H, Kohane IS. Framing the challenges of artificial intelligence in medicine. BMJ Qual Saf 2019;28(3):238–41.
34. Kim Y-E, Ki C-S, Jang M-A. Challenges and considerations in sequence variant interpretation for mendelian disorders. Ann Lab Med 2019;39(5):421.
35. Schwab AP, Luu HS, Wang J, et al. Genomic privacy. Clin Chem 2018;64(12): 1696–703.
36. Gerke S, Babic B, Evgeniou T, et al. The need for a system view to regulate artificial intelligence/machine learning-based software as medical device. NPJ Digit Med 2020;3(1):53.
37. Zook JM, McDaniel J, Olson ND, et al. An open resource for accurately benchmarking small variant and reference calls. Nat Biotechnol 2019;37(5):561–6.
38. Bodenreider O. The Unified Medical Language System (UMLS): integrating biomedical terminology. Nucleic Acids Res 2004;32(Database issue):D267–70.
39. DePristo MA, Banks E, Poplin R, et al. A framework for variation discovery and genotyping using next-generation DNA sequencing data. Nat Genet 2011; 43(5):491–8.
40. Gelman A, Carlin JB, Stern HS, et al. Bayesian data analysis. 3rd edition. Chapman and Hall/CRC Press Taylor and Francis Group; 2013.
41. Schriml LM, Mitraka E, Munro J, et al. Human Disease Ontology 2018 update: classification, content and workflow expansion. Nucleic Acids Res 2019; 47(D1):D955–62.
42. Köhler S, Carmody L, Vasilevsky N, et al. Expansion of the Human Phenotype Ontology (HPO) knowledge base and resources. Nucleic Acids Res 2019; 47(D1):D1018–27.
43. World Health Organization. ICD-10: international statistical classification of diseases and related health problems/World Health Organization. 10th revision, 2nd edition. Geneva (Switzerland): World Health Organization; 2004.
44. McKusick-Nathans Institute of Genetic Medicine. Online Mendelian Inheritance in Man, OMIM®. [Internet]. Available at: https://omim.org/. Accessed January 1, 2020.
45. Cornet R, de Keizer N. Forty years of SNOMED: a literature review. BMC Med Inform Decis Mak 2008;8(Suppl 1):S2.
46. Mungall CJ, McMurry JA, Köhler S, et al. The Monarch Initiative: an integrative data and analytic platform connecting phenotypes to genotypes across species. Nucleic Acids Res 2017;45(D1):D712–22.

Moving?

Make sure your subscription moves with you!

To notify us of your new address, find your **Clinics Account Number** (located on your mailing label above your name), and contact customer service at:

Email: journalscustomerservice-usa@elsevier.com

800-654-2452 (subscribers in the U.S. & Canada)
314-447-8871 (subscribers outside of the U.S. & Canada)

Fax number: 314-447-8029

Elsevier Health Sciences Division
Subscription Customer Service
3251 Riverport Lane
Maryland Heights, MO 63043

Moving?

Make sure your subscription
moves with you!

To notify us of your new address, find your Clinics Account
number (located on your mailing label above your name),
and contact customer service at:

Email: journalscustomerservice-usa@elsevier.com

800-654-2452 (subscribers in the U.S. & Canada)
314-447-8871 (subscribers outside of the U.S. & Canada)

Fax number: 314-447-8029

Elsevier Health Sciences Division
Subscription Customer Service
3251 Riverport Lane
Maryland Heights, MO 63043

To ensure uninterrupted delivery of your subscription,
please notify us at least 4 weeks in advance of move.

Printed and bound by CPI Group (UK) Ltd, Croydon, CR0 4YY

03/10/2024

01040473-0013